The Alzheimer's or Memory Café

How to Start and Succeed with Your Own Café

Jytte Fogh Lokvig, Ph.D.

Endless Circle Press

ISBN: 9780971039087

Prepublication Edition: August 1, 2016

LIBRARY OF CONGRESS CONTROL NUMBER: Pending

Endless Circle Press
228 Ojo de la Vaca Rd.
Santa Fe, NM 87508
(505)466-8195
Email: ECP@gmail.com

Other books by Dr. Jytte Lokvig, Ph.D.
  Alzheimer's A to Z, Secrets to Successful Caregiving
  Alzheimer's A to Z, A Quick Reference Guide
  The Alzheimer's Creativity Project
  Alzheimer's and Dementia Handbook

Contents

Chapter Eight

Chapter Nine

Chapter Ten

Chapter Eleven

Acknowledgments

Special thanks to Thresa Grady for believing in the mission of the Alzheimer's and Memory Café movement, your patience and steadfast support of this book project and to Bioclinica for their sponsorship.

The Alzheimer's and Memory Cafés have brought together a nationwide network of amazing, creative, and selfless people, among the early pioneers, Paula Rais, Carole Larkin, Gary Glazner, Cecily Kaplan, and Carin Mack; Maryann Frantz, Debora Tingley, and Lori La Bey, as well as Susan and John McFadden.

In preparing this book, I've had so many wonderful conversations with many of you who lead your own cafés. Every one of you told me that the Café is one of the best projects you've ever taken on and you all expressed how you wanted to see this concept spread far and wide. Thank you to the many of you, who have generously and enthusiastically shared your thoughts and ideas.

Thank you to my colleagues and friends, who took the time to review and give me input on the manuscript. Thank you for catching the missing commas and other edits to Emily Freede, Kairand Bellinger, Jan Olsen, and Terry Lee Morris.

The café in Santa Fe owes its success to a strong core of participants, some living with dementia, others friends of the cafe, among them Sandra Oppenheimer, Heather Darden, Suki Groseclose, Jan Olsen, and Sue Foley. More recently Roxanne Brie and Susan Balkman.

Author

Dr. Jytte Fogh Lokvig

Lokvig introduced the Alzheimer's Café concept to the United States, when she opened the café in Santa Fe, NM in 2008. Since then she has guided numerous other communities to start their own cafés. In 2012 she set up the original national registry of cafés to help people locate cafés in their own communities.

Jytte Lokvig grew up in Copenhagen, Denmark. After coming to this country as a young adult, she attended the Art Center College of Design in Los Angeles and later earned her degrees at Antioch College/West, California State University at Los Angeles, and California Pacific University, where she earned a doctoral degree in management, specializing in Alzheimer's and dementia caregiving.

Lokvig has long been at the forefront of social change. She was among the founding parent group and later a teacher at the first publicly funded alternative in southern California. This pilot program introduced humanistic approaches to education in the greater Los Angeles school district. She designed and led the school's successful art program. Based on a center model, she was able to offer a wide array of arts and crafts skills while allowing students to work at their own pace and follow their own passions.

With an extensive art and design career, Lokvig has designed costumes for stage and screen as well as for her own boutique in Hollywood. Her fine arts works have shown internationally. For over a decade, she was active in The Women's Caucus for Art, a nationwide advocacy movement to promote inclusion of women in the professional arts. She headed up the special events and exhibitions for the group, served as president of the Southern California chapter and was a member of the national steering committee. Under the auspices of the WCA, she produced and hosted a television series featuring women artists.

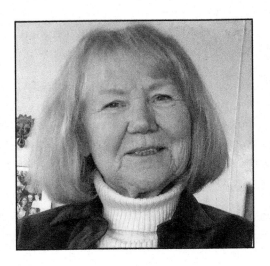

Jytte left Los Angeles in 1988 for Santa Fe, New Mexico. Here she was introduced to a large community of elders living with dementia, mostly Alzheimer's. Since then, she has devoted herself to improving the lives of people living with dementia as well as their families and caregivers, including authoring several books on communication, creativity and caregiving. She is frequently invited to speak on successful caregiving, as well as a counselor for caregivers and people living with cognitive impairment.

Foreword

Loneliness and lack of purpose are two primary reasons for shortened lifespans as well as depression in older adults. Thanks to the work of people like Tom Kitwood, Bill Thomas, MD and Al Power, MD, we're realizing that both issues are also responsible for hastened decline in cognition in folks living with dementia, including Alzheimer's. These disorders make it harder for the individual to initiate contacts, conversations, or purposeful projects. Loneliness is not limited to physical isolation; the worst kind of lonely is the alienation you feel when you're in the middle of a crowd, but deprived of connections and purpose.

If you're involved with the cognitive-impairment community, I'm sure you're always on the lookout for something to help your care partners live well with dementia. I was struck with relief and excitement when I discovered the Alzheimer's Café concept. Now, after years of witnessing the success of hundreds of cafés around the country, I decided it was time to share this information with as many of you as possible.

This book takes you through the simple steps to start your own café and as I have, I trust you'll discover that this is one of your most effective endeavors ever.

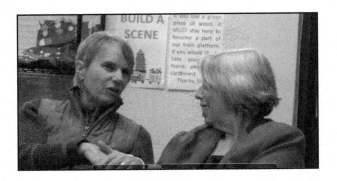

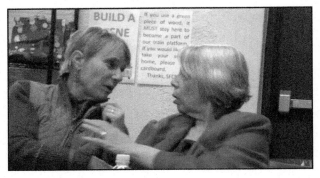

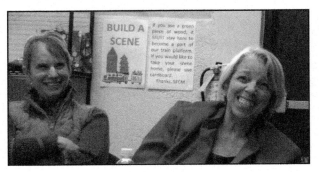

Chapter One

Introduction

The Alzheimer's Café is the best project I've ever taken on, the simplest and most natural way to bring joy to those who are living with dementia as well as their caregivers and families. With a space, a few snacks, something fun and creative to do, sing-alongs, word games, or simply conversations, you can have a profound impact on your guests.

Our Alzheimer's Café in Santa Fe has been going strong since its inception in 2008. Ours is a modest little program that has been bringing joy, emotional respite, and relief to our numerous guests over the years. Whether we have two guests or fifteen, we focus on fun and companionship.

We've had as many as twenty-seven guests, crammed in like sardines and as few as *one*, but somehow it was always just exactly right. The large group enjoyed a rousing sing-along; on the other hand our single guest really needed to talk about sensitive issues.

In early 2008, on one of my regular online searches, my eyes caught a new item: "Alzheimer's <u>Café</u>." It was an instant "lightbulb" moment: goose bumps and a light head. Much to the consternation of my cat, who'd been snoozing at my feet, out loud I exclaimed, "WOW! I'LL BE! – *WHY DIDN'T I THINK OF THAT?*"

In that moment, I knew this might be the answer I had long sought for a way to bring together people living with dementia

1

and their loved ones in a setting that allows everyone to relax and enjoy each others company, free of the pressures that a cognitive disorder brings to all daily interactions, tasks and responsibilities. I knew how special it can be to share joyful moments with a person living with Alzheimer's and I also knew that many people never get the opportunity to have those precious experiences. Many of our family members have confirmed how the café has changed their relationships and the demeanor of their loved ones. One wife told how the café had 'given her back the husband who had been absent since his dementia had taken over.' She thanked us profusely for the chance to once again see the man she had married, full of joy and confidence.

NOTE: I may use the term: *Alzheimer's Café* or simply *The Café*, to represent any café, whether it's known as an Alzheimer's Café, a Memory Café, or any other name.

What is an Alzheimer's or Memory Café?

The Alzheimer's Café is a very simple concept, a monthly gathering in a friendly space where people living with dementia and their caregivers can relax and form friendships for mutual support. The Café gives people with dementia the opportunity to share a positive experience with their companions, a chance to explore art, music, poetry and socialization. Laughter, companionship, and love are the keystones of these cafés.

> "One of the essential ingredients of the Café is that care partners and people dealing with the disease have an enjoyable outing together. The Café provides an informal place to find out how others deal with the illness and its consequences. The low threshold environment allows visitors to feel at home, talk informally, and find recognition and acceptance."
>
> Paula Rais, Dover, NH

> "I think a lot of times people think about Alzheimer's disease as such a negative and depressing thing, and it does not have to be that way. When people come to a Memory Café, it's such an uplifting experience for people to realize, 'Hey, I can still contribute something.'"
>
> April Stauffer, KY

When Doctor Miesen started his initial project in 1997, he could have called it a *club*, a *meeting*, or a *group*, but he chose the term Café deliberately to suggest the informal nature of a public café. A Café is an informal public venue that requires no reservations. People can drop in for a quick cup of coffee or stay for long conversations with friends. Thus the Alzheimer's Café is

3

a social event with an open invitation to everybody involved with Alzheimer's or other dementias. Ironically, despite the name, The Alzheimer's Café offers respite from the pressures and burdens of the disease.

Alzheimer's Cafés vary in name and structure, but all the groups share some essential characteristics that commonly define them:

- A regularly scheduled gathering of people with dementia AND their caregivers and other people in their lives

- A safe, supportive, and engaging environment.

- A non–judgmental atmosphere

- A meeting place that is warm, comfortable, and friendly

- No reservations required: The casual structure allows participants to attend on a drop-in basis

- Enough unstructured time to allow mingling and conversation

- Something interesting to do, a fun activity of some sort, preferably something creative

- Some simple food and drink

- A place for the caregiver and person with dementia to interact with each other in new ways

- A place to make new friends, share stories, including feelings about the challenges of living with dementia

Most cafés meet monthly, preferably in a location not associated with elder or medical care. The idea is to promote social interaction and provide respite from daily routines that are too often dementia-centric. The café gives participants (café guests) an opportunity to share a positive experience, often by exploring art, music and poetry.

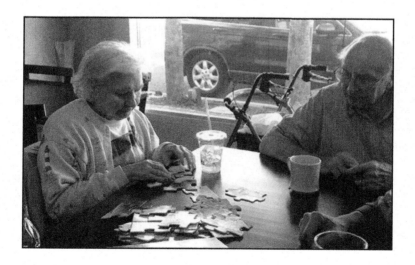

What it is not

- The Alzheimer's Café is <u>not</u> adult daycare

- It's not a promotion for any cause or business (we do not display pamphlets or other advertising)

- It's not respite care, a place for caregivers to drop-off someone who needs care and supervision

- Although the Café is a supportive environment, it is <u>not</u> a support group

- The focus is on social activity and creative expression, rather than problem-solving and education

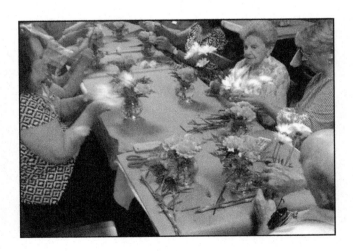

6

A Special Event

Beth Soltzberg has been successful in organizing several cafés in the Boston area. She calls her program "The Percolator." She tells of how a woman, attending with her husband who's living with Alzheimer's, expressed her relief at finding the café. She said, "There is definitely a role for adult day health and other more formal programs. But my husband has so much life in him and those programs can be very passive. This, for us, is so much more invigorating and hopeful. This café is really the best news I've had since he was diagnosed."

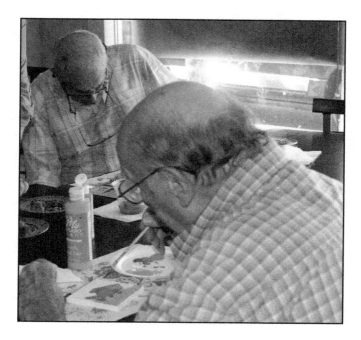

Beth adds, "What's better than having a cup of coffee and enjoying some music with a friend? It may seem like a simple pleasure, but for people living with dementia, it can be a rare one. With memory changes, life becomes about what you can't do. For a person who doesn't have dementia to see their partner laughing can recharge that relationship. We don't focus on disease. We focus on life and helping people connect."

At the Alzheimer's Café, the caregiver and the person with dementia participate together.

"Unlike a caregiver support group, respite or adult day program, an Alzheimer's Café model engages people affected by the disease and their care partners together in a social setting. We wanted to provide a safe, supportive and judgment-free setting where care partners and those affected by the disease could enjoy an afternoon in the company of people on the same journey. With the help of volunteers who welcome visitors and keep everyone engaged in conversation, we hoped that families would feel comfortable, calm and happy, make new friends and discover helpful resources."

Paula Rais, NH

Hope Matters is Maryann Makekau's creation and her focus. Through writing, speaking and advocacy, she spreads love and hope to people coping with cancer, deployment in war, dementia and other difficult life situations. Where memory loss is concerned, it's personal – her mother is living with Alzheimer's. Maryann is a caregiver for both her parents, and in many ways for others walking in her shoes.

"The holidays conjure up images of family and friends gathered around the table, feasting on turkey and all the fixings, engaged in jovial conversation before migrating to the living room to watch the football game. Much like those holiday gatherings, I had envisioned a public place that replicated a sense of the family meal. Too often families going through Alzheimer's or other types of dementia are isolated. Venturing out of the home or care facility to attend a gathering can be a source of stress when the destination is not user-friendly.

So, I created a co-op where worry and anxiety are eased and love and hope are tangible. The come-as-you-are "neighborhood memory cafes" are a place with handicap accessibility from parking and entry to restroom facilities (wipes, gloves, and briefs included). Caregivers and their loved ones enjoy a "family meal" while immersing in various forms of art, table-side. Volunteers help me with the details and sponsors cover related costs such as refreshments and visiting artists.

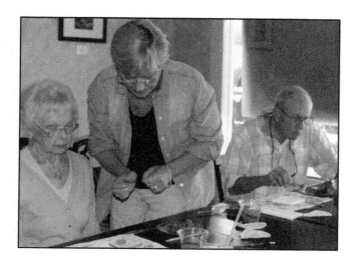

Meals out, indulgence in the arts, and lively conversations are unfortunately rare treats. Together we can change that; let's push back against the stereotypes surrounding dementia. Love comes in many forms for those "stuck inside" dementia affected bodies and their decade-plus caregivers. Let us be love in motion. That tops my holiday wish list. How about yours?

Two neighborhood memory cafés operate on a monthly basis, and now a third has been set in motion. When one of our venues closed for renovation, my mother's care center volunteered to host it. The gathering brought an overwhelmingly positive response. Now, the activities director is committed to hosting a monthly café for the families they serve. That demonstrates a contagious quality I had hoped for my community. The National Registry of Alzheimer's Cafes lists hundreds of locations along with an online tool kit."

Maryann Makekau, FL

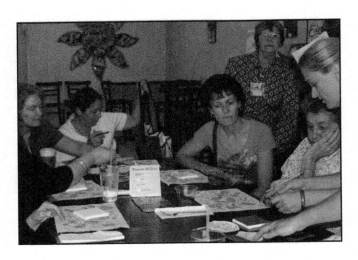

History of the Alzheimer's Café

The Alzheimer's Café is the brainchild Dr. Bere Miesen, a Dutch geriatric psychiatrist. He had a growing frustration with the medical establishment's increasing reliance on pharmaceutical remedies at the expense of people's emotional and social needs.

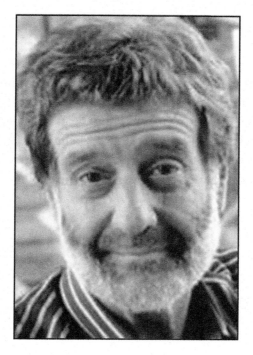

Dr. Miesen was convinced that the issues involved in having and living with dementia needed to be discussed openly and where better to do this than in an open, friendly environment like a casual neighborhood café? His first café in 1997 drew around 30 people, but with subsequent cafés the number of guests grew so quickly that he started a second café, then another and another as the needs dictated. By late 2015 there were over 200 cafés in the Netherlands, a nation the size of the state of Maryland.

In the year 2000, Dr. Miesen and Dr. Gemma Jones introduced the Alzheimer Café into the United Kingdom, where the movement continues to expand. Later some communities in Britain started calling their events "memory" café.

The café concept has quickly spread throughout Europe and jumped across the "pond" when I started the Alzheimer's Café in Santa Fe, New Mexico. The movement is now growing worldwide. I believe that in another ten years, the Alzheimer's Cafés will be as commonplace in our communities as libraries and other community venues and we'll wonder how we ever managed without them.

Chapter Two

A Café in Every Community

The Alzheimer's (and Memory) Café movement is growing and public perception is slowly changing from the café being a novelty to a staple in many communities. The café is a safe and judgment-free environment that gives everyone a respite from the constant emotional turmoil brought on by dementia. Many families and caregivers have reported to us the delight in the positive changes in their loved ones. One wife was astonished when her husband joined our sing-along with enthusiasm and a big grin on his face. She hadn't heard him sing in several years and she had rarely seen him smile.

The café gives everyone a break from the pressures dementia puts on their daily lives. Finally there's a place out in public where nobody flinches if a word or gesture comes out wrong. When families and caregivers share these experiences it helps them see the individual living with dementia with fresh eyes. Here the typical expressions of dementia, forgetting names, words, how to do things, are simply the norm and everyone accepts the occasional bumps as par for the course. The person living with Alzheimer's or related dementia can relax and feel "normal" out in public.

Filling a Need

Loneliness and lack of purpose are particularly difficult for folks living with dementia, including Alzheimer's. These disorders make it harder for the individual to initiate contacts, conversations, or purposeful projects.

Loneliness is not limited to physical isolation; the worst kind of lonely is the alienation you feel when you're in the middle of a crowd, but deprived of connections and purpose.

"For over a decade now, I have been loving my parents through Mom's battle with Alzheimer's. First as a long-distance caregiver while my sisters championed support. Then, almost two years ago, my husband and I assumed the role of close-up caregivers. There are millions of others, just like us, around the nation. According to The MetLife Study of Working Caregivers and Employer Healthcare Costs there are nearly 10 million adult children older than 50 who are caring for aging parents.

So, who is caring for the caregivers? Alzheimer's and other forms of dementia often require 7-10 years of caregiving support. Burnout, depression, and isolation are common ripple effects of the very demanding unpaid work. In an effort to reframe the tough journey for caregivers, as well as those living with dementia, I launched a Neighborhood Memory Cafe last summer; and a second one is set to open next week. The monthly gatherings include some perks:

entertainment, healthy snacks, and a safe place for caregivers to enjoy quality time with their loved ones."

Maryann Makenau, FL

Humans are social beings with a fundamental need to feel part of the community and to be able to contribute in some way. It's not natural for us to be idle. Not having purpose can be isolating and detrimental to our wellbeing. Unfortunately this may happen even when a person lives in a long-term care community, many of which offer little in the way of stimulating projects or purposeful engagement.

"This weekend, a customer came in while I was working a shift. After I introduced myself as the "manager," he proceeded to tell me how thankful he was for Memory Café. He mentioned that his parents recently started attending as his mother's dementia has gotten worse. He indicated that she is very self-conscious about her memory issues, but she has been warmly welcomed at Memory Café. He also mentioned that his dad is very introverted but has loved his experience at Memory Café. Finally, he asked me to pass on his thanks because it has become the highlight of his parents' week! Just wanted to pass that along! . . . Yay Memory Café!!"

Nikki at J. Arthur's Coffee Shop, MN

Fighting the Stigma

Tom Hlavacek calls the opening of a Memory Café in Greendale momentous. He's executive director of the Alzheimer's Association of Southeastern Wisconsin.

> "People with Alzheimer's and their care partners are pulling this disease out of the shadows and they're saying no more! No more are we going to live a life of stigma, no more are we going to live a life of stereotyping."
>
> Tom Hlavacek, WI

The Greendale café is located at Ferch's Malt Shoppe. It will host social events for people with dementia and their care givers, such as games and music.
One person who plans to visit is Wayne Klopfer; his wife was diagnosed with Alzheimer's two years ago.

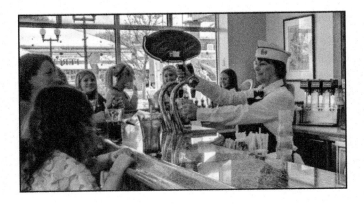

"There's a fellow named Tim and he's a good singer and he brings along sheets of Seeger. He gets going on a pitch pipe and we'll sing Christmas carols and kids coming walking in and joining us," Klopfer says and adds that he's pleased the new Memory Café is closer to home.

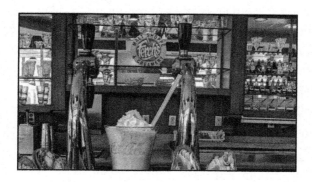

Another person who came to the official opening is Bashir Easter of the Milwaukee County Department on Aging. His mother has been living with Alzheimer's for 11 years. Easter says Memory Cafés support the caregivers too, so he's happy for his sister and mom. "I encourage my sister, who is her caregiver, to get out. The Memory Café is not just for the individual who has the disease, it's also for the caregiver, to give them a break and we see that in these cafes," Easter says.

Isolation and loneliness can be equally present for people who live at home with family or a caregiver. More often than not, their daily lives are focused on dementia-related issues and their only contacts with the outside world are trips to doctors' offices. A few families have been fortunate enough to meet others in their situation and have collaborated to support each other. Some of these efforts have grown out of relationships started at an Alzheimer's or Memory Café.

"Another interesting encounter at the Dementia Café lunch meet yesterday. A friend brought her mother who had recently come to live with her. Someone with possible early dementia or just stress-related issues. When she asked if she should bring her mother, I'd encouraged it strongly but suggested she didn't specifically say it was a dementia support lunch. Just call it a social occasion.

It worked so well. Very social, very relaxed. Mom obviously enjoyed it and chatted with the others. This also means that, if her daughter needed extra contact with help later, her Mom would already feel at home with those folks.

To me, with years of facilitating support groups*, I'm thinking to myself "DUH!". It was always so obvious it should be this way. Thank goodness we are waking up."

Frena Gray-Davidson, AZ

*The majority of support groups focus on problems encountered by caregivers. The groups rarely address issues brought up by those living with dementia. Thus by their nature they are one-sided and tend to be mostly focused on the negative.

Living with Dementia

There's a general misconception that memory-impairment is simply "forgetting" where you can retrieve your thoughts later, as in: "It'll come to you. Just relax." Memory-impairment due to dementia is more than that. Some of my clients, who are living with dementia, describe it as a bottomless black hole; the more you try, the deeper the hole. In other words, it's simply gone. They tell me about being in what should be a familiar situation or location and not recognizing anything. This explains why some people cannot find their way home to a place where they've lived for a decade. No wonder this arouses fear in the general public. The tendency often is to retreat and avoid contact with people with these disorders. Sadly, many so-called friends withdraw and vanish into the woodwork.

A good friend and a powerful spokesperson for living well with dementia was the late Dr. Richard Taylor. He had been given a diagnosis of Alzheimer's three years prior to making it public, but had decided to keep it to himself. People around him during that time were blissfully unaware. Once he revealed his diagnosis, he found himself suddenly isolated, no more phone calls, no invitations, and no impromptu visits from his wide circle of friends and acquaintances. After a few weeks of silence and realizing that he was at risk for depression, he called several of them to find out "why this silence." One after another said they didn't know how to talk to him and were afraid of saying something wrong. He reminded them that they had none of those problems when they had conversations just weeks ago, the diagnosis had not changed who he was.

Few people have the strength and self-assurance of Dr. Richard Taylor. Many give in to the isolation and become withdrawn. Being out in public is particularly stressful. Some may feel shunned as their behavior appears more unconventional. Progressively the contacts with the outside world are limited to those of necessity, typically medical appointments. This obviously leads to increased isolation for both those living with dementia and their caregivers.

The Alzheimer's Café is the one occasion when people can be themselves. The care partners can talk openly about their daily lives, frustrations and joys alike. The café is a non-judgmental environment of mutual support without actually being a formal "support group." Interestingly, at our cafe, the topics around dementia or caregiving hardly ever come up and when they do, they get the same attention as any other discussion. Sometimes we talk about our dogs, our grandchildren, or our childhoods. Or we may talk about losing the sense of smell, sensitivity to noise, or troubles with speech. This aura of normalcy has always been an important aspect of our cafe.

"Joe has been coming home very enthused about some of the discussions, and I think it's helped him acknowledge that he has Alzheimer's because at first he was in denial. I think he thought of it as being a stigma. He didn't want people to even know. Now it's more like it's OK."

Marlene Straughan. KY

Memory Cafés for All

An Experiment. By Beth Soltzberg, Boston, Massachusetts

One growing population of people living with dementia is those who also have a developmental disability. People with developmental disabilities are living longer than ever before so many are now developing dementia and people with Down syndrome and traumatic brain injury have a particularly high risk of developing a condition that causes dementia as they age. We applaud the Massachusetts Department of Developmental Services (DDS) for being the first in the nation to support the launch of memory cafés that are designed to include people with dementia who also have developmental disabilities. DDS is offering seed funding to new cafés working toward this goal.

In response, I have been leading trainings on starting a memory café around Massachusetts in collaboration with DDS. DDS leaders recognize that truly including those who have dementia plus a developmental disability requires more than just saying that the café is open to all; it requires collaboration between aging and disabilities service providers as well as listening to the true experts – those living with dementia. There are barriers: professionals from these two service systems have different funding sources and ways of serving clients, and quite simply, often don't know each other. While memory cafés have always worked to end stigma towards those living with dementia, they now must grapple with the stigma that exists toward those with developmental disabilities as well. This is hard work. There is no one more capable of doing it, though,

21

than people who have spent their careers advocating for full inclusion of people with disabilities and older adults.

In addition to striving to make all memory cafés truly accessible and responsive to the wide variety of people with dementia, it is exciting to see the seeds of new cafés that are embedded in particular cultural communities. For example, we hope to see the launch of the first Spanish-speaking memory cafés this year.

While people living with Alzheimer's or related disorders may share a diagnosis that shapes their life and the life of the people who are close to them in many similar ways, they remain unique individuals with their own culture, personality, and developmental needs. These aspects of who they are don't go away with a diagnosis; in fact, they may become more important than ever. Memory cafés in Massachusetts are working to respond. Because for all of us, there's no place like home.

Beth Soltzberg's "Percolator" supports
many cafés in the Boston area

Confetti, a Poem

Stuart Hall lived with an undetermined dementia. He was prolific poet, or "wordsmith" as he preferred to call himself. According to his wife, he averaged thirty poems a day, scribbled on any scrap of paper within reach. The following is his 'take' on living with dementia:

My mind's not at all a blank slate,
Though I cannot keep track of the date
    Or the day of the week,
    And facts play hide-and-seek,
For my mind to be blank would be great.

Instead, it is wired like spaghetti;
It conflates the important and petty;
    The connections of things
    Are like tangles of strings
Or like celebratory confetti.

Stuart Hall, NM

Living with a progressive cognitive disorder is stressful for everyone involved. Persons living with the disease may be aware of their abilities slipping, with sudden gaps in their short-term memory, losing control of their lives and feeling alienated from those around them. Family members and friends have a difficult time coping and understanding that their loved ones still look the same, but are slowly changing from the people they used to know. Few of us are prepared for these changes, which can lead to conflict, depression, and anxiety.

Las Vegas, NV

BooksorBooks Bookstore in Las Vegas hosts a unique Alzheimer's Café started by Nancy Nelson, an author and poet, who is living with Alzheimer's.

"Every other month I organize a local author book signing at our community-oriented BooksorBooks Bookstore. Diagnosed with Alzheimer's disease (AD) and living with the changes taking place in my brain since 2013, I have a bit of experience in plowing my way through the sadness, fear, and frustration that this horrific disease causes. Sharing these poems is a way to show insights about someone living well with the AD diagnosis, speaking out, building awareness, reducing stigma, and to advocate with elected officials on key legislative priorities.

We sit and talk in a relaxed environment where everyone can learn, find friendship, and revel in the peace and wisdom shared within the walls of this truly wonderful family bookstore shelving over 30,000 books. Perhaps, we are all sharing in baby steps to a bigger and more comprehensive Alzheimer's Café one day.

It is sure gratifying, the feeling that collectively we are making a difference. My grandmother would say, "Many hands make light work." Smiling at the thought of her saying it; and today knowing, how true… I cherish being surrounded by dear friends and their willingness to help in all endeavors, I'm blessed."

Nancy Nelson, NV

Blue. River. *Apple.*
by Nancy Nelson

I know I have done it again!

Do I *stay home, cancel, quit?*
Or *fight for right of passage through the fog?*
Silently. I say. I am not what I appear.
Times mix up, promises go astray.
When I hear, "Where are you?" "Are you coming?"
Eyes water, stomach churns, humbled in disbelief.

Breathe in courage

Struggle to remember . . .

I am sorry for what you see.
Chin up treading lightly in new uncharted waters.

At times, I catch sideways glances, back-and-forth.
Perhaps, even, your voice impatient. I *understand.*
Splash on the smile,

I must find pieces of myself and revel in who I know I am.
But, wait, we stand together, separate.
Can you hear me? I have so much to tell you.

I am Warrior

Garage door grinds shut.

Did I forget to close it?

- Sssh, sleep, it is okay.

I lay awake
Fear re-surfaces
Inner tunnels of my mind ...

Did I leave our house unprotected?

- Sssh, sleep.

Night passes.
Do I ask or lay silent?
Warrior or Coward?
Eyes close, I snuggle in.
No decision is a decision.
Wrong choice, Warrior.

Prepared to do better
But, caught in between ...
Did I? Or didn't I?
Please help me...remember.

Go ahead,

Take a chance, ask.

"Son, did I forget to close the garage door?"
"No, Mom, I came in late."

Remember, Warrior,
Always ask.
Stand tall, straight and accountable
Again.

My shoulders square,
My jaw relaxes.
My heart sings!
I am who I want to be

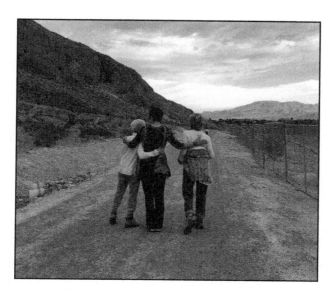

Purpose

Susan is a retired therapist, outgoing, compassionate, and friendly. When I first met her, she had been living for a couple of years with a diagnosis of younger-onset dementia, probably of the Alzheimer's type. At our first meeting, she tearfully talked about her increasing feeling of alienation from her family and friends. She had tried to convey to them how the world was changing for her and to explain her fears, feelings and experiences to them. Rather than attempt to understand, they would react with, "we all forget sometimes" or they would present a variety of 'logical' explanations, all in the belief that this would reassure her.

Her well-meaning family and friends didn't realize that rather than reassuring Susan, these consistent denials of her feelings were dismissing her instead, as though she couldn't possibly know better than them. In trying to convey that 'we're in this together' her friends were achieving just the opposite.

In their defense, it's a normal reaction for us to want to make our friends feel better, so we try to reassure them that this "boo– boo" will get better.

However, dementia does not get better

After half an hour into our meeting, Susan wiped her tears and we started to talking about how to go forward. She told me about her worries and her pleasures. Several of her old routines were now affected by the dementia. It was particularly hard to know she'd have to give up her practice as a therapist. We then explored what could give her new purpose. She told me that over the years, she'd enjoyed sporadic sessions at Santa Fe Clay.

Her eyes lit up again as she talked about making this her new mission. Since then, Susan's pottery has become her vocation. She now shows and sells her pottery at local art fairs and shows.

Later she told me that this had been a good decision. Santa Fe Clay is a large ceramics studio with several potters, giving Susan companionship with folks who shared her love for the craft. She found that working on the wheel also was ideal by giving her the extra time that she might need to get her thoughts together. And when she wasn't sure of herself, it is the perfect excuse not to respond to questions,. Everyone in the studio understands that there are times 'when our work requires our full attention.'

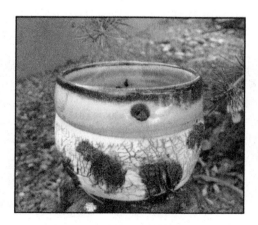

One of Susan's creations

"The biggest change for me since having dementia, is that my language was beginning to diminish so much that I found myself not talking, preferring instead being silent. When people asked me a question, I could not get the words out or I could not remember how to speak. Taking up pottery has changed my life. I have something that I love to do. Now after 2 years, my language expression is better, not totally back, and there are still many moments when I am in what I call la la land when someone is talking to me. Yet, more often, I can carry a conversation for a while before anyone could tell that something is not quite right; that I'm struggling for the words or not being able to remember what something. My ability to speak, being able to form words, and speak them clearly has begun to improve.

The other important aspect of working creatively is my coordination is better and my self-confidence has improved."

Susan Balkman

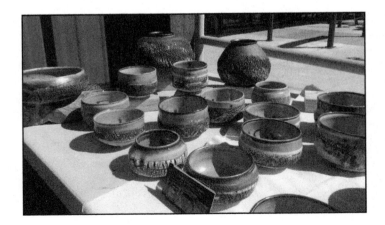

Chapter Three

Starting Your Own Café:

- A venue with a warm and inviting atmosphere, not too big and not too small, preferably FREE

- Accessible, ample parking

- Comfortable furniture (We prefer a single oversized table with enough chairs for all our guests)

- A host with experience with Alzheimer's and dementia and a group of people dedicated to the idea that people with dementia deserve to enjoy life as much as anyone else

- A modest spread of snacks, fruits, and drinks

- Supplies for projects

- Contact people with Alzheimer's or dementia and their caregivers, friends or family

- Contact Alzheimer's support groups, senior centers, medical offices, and others who have regular contact with elders

- Contact local media. If you have a local radio station, ask them to invite you to talk about your café

Choosing Your Venue

The Café gives everyone a break from the focus on the disease. It starts with setting up your Café in a warm and inviting environment where everyone feels safe to be himself or herself. Most of the current café leaders recommend choosing a venue that's not too big and not too small, with comfortable furniture, good lighting, and good acoustics. Most cafés are held in rent-free venues, so they can offer the program at no charge or for a minimal donation. Some cafés take place in coffee shops and actual cafés, where the only expense is the cost of their individual orders.

Many cafés prefer locations with no specific association with the medical community or with a service for elders or seniors. Some examples of café locations include Restaurants, ice cream parlors, coffee shops, children's museums, art museums, theaters, libraries, community centers.

> "Our café met for the first two months in a senior daycare center, but the opportunity arose to meet regularly in a local coffee shop. It has been one of the best things we've done, as people really seem to like the atmosphere of the coffee shop, and it makes it feel like a "date" for some of our married couples. The mission-minded coffee shop has a great menu and we encourage attendees to purchase refreshments. Because of this change to support the coffee shop, we can now allocate more money to Memory Café programming, rather than food and beverage for the group."
>
> Allison Sawyer, GA

One of the primary purposes of the café is for care partners to get away from their usual routines and locations and get out into the community at large. Thus venues of last resort are those associated with elders or caregiving, such as senior centers, care facilities, nursing homes, medical facilities, or adult daycare centers. If you have no other option than to offer your café in a senior center or a care facility, it's important that your café stands apart from other activities and is NOT treated as simply another *happy hour.* All efforts should be made to open your cafe to the community as well as to bring in families and friends of the local residents.

"Look for a place that will accommodate the special needs of this group: Choosing a place that feels comfortable and safe ideally will include being tucked away from high traffic areas, with the option of a back-door entry, if warranted. It should also be amenable to transfers in and out of a car, and bathrooms that aren't just accessible, but roomy, so caregivers can escort their loved one.

Provide quiet spaces or soothing familiar tunes: Noise can over-stimulate those living with dementia, so look for quiet spaces. One of the host cafés added a curtain and quieting ceiling panels to create an intimate feeling. They also utilize a sound system and pipe in favorite tunes through Pandora Radio."

Maryann Makekau, FL

Venue Search in Santa Fe

We consider ourselves very fortunate that our Alzheimer's Café has a "home" at the Children's Museum in Santa Fe.

It took a couple of detours to get here.

When I set out to start our project, I felt it would be important for us to be in a "neutral" space, not associated with any medical or eldercare institutions or particular religious denominations. I looked at coffee shops and cafés, big and small; I was a little leery about a public venue like a coffee shop, since I had no way of knowing who would show up. I had years of experience with dementia populations at various stages of the disease, so I knew that I would have to be prepared for any eventuality. I would be fine with that, but I wasn't sure other patrons in a restaurant would be quite as understanding.

I considered a couple of private homes, but there were problems with access, parking, and stairs. A couple of libraries offered the use of their meeting rooms, but they didn't allow food and drinks, so we couldn't have snacks and with no running water, we also wouldn't be able to paint or use clay. After three months, I was offered a meeting room at the College of Santa Fe. It looked like a club and turned out to be perfect for the first several meetings, which drew unusually large crowds. By the fourth café our attendance was more modest, making the space feel a little too big and a bit too "stuffy" to be comfortable, so we started looking around again. Good thing!

Timing could not have been better. We had just arranged to use the community room in a senior apartment complex when we got word that the College of Santa Fe had ceased to exist. A year later the college was to become the Santa Fe University of Art and Design. The community room was adequate, had great lighting, decent parking, and a nice view, but it was a bit impersonal and since it was used by the senior lunch program an hour before we'd arrive, it always had a faint hint of wet oilcloth table covers.

I decided to look for a new location. Santa Fe is home to many beautiful museums that all have community rooms, but one after the other quoted rents that were way out of reach for us. Fate stepped in when I met a woman who used to work at the Santa Fe Children's Museum. She got me an appointment with the director. As luck had it, the director had a very soft heart for dementia; his beloved grandmother had lived with Alzheimer's. All through college he had spent most of his weekends with her. He was so excited about our project and I was so thrilled to meet someone who got the purpose of the café. We had talked over each other to the point that I had to ask the assistant who'd been standing by what we had decided. We've been there ever since. There's something special about being in a children's museum. Even when we're in a classroom separate from the museum activities, we'll still hear delighted squeals of little kids and occasionally a little one will wander into the room. We have an open invitation to explore the museum when our participants want to take a break.

Choosing Day and Time

The Alzheimer Cafés in Britain started by meeting in late afternoons and early evenings. They soon realized that their meeting times were in direct competition with televised soccer games and other popular after-work activities, so they switched to daytime programs.

Our café meets the second Wednesday of the month from 2 to 4 pm in the afternoon. This timing is quite deliberate. 2 pm is after lunch and 4 pm precedes dinner and dusk. (Many caregivers are elderly and don't like to drive in the dark.) We have an open invitation to the community at large. Our set schedule and fixed location allow people to drop in with no advance notice.

Choosing the second week of the month was also deliberate, since many of our guests belong to a demographic that still relies on old-fashioned wall calendars and many people forget to turn the page to the new month until the second week.

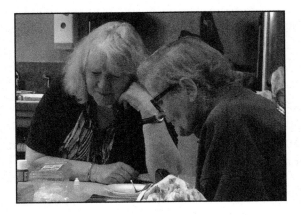

Association or Not

Several cafés in the United States are sponsored by organizations, care facilities, and home care providers. When I started our cafe in Santa Fe, I had no idea where we would be going or what to expect, so I felt it was important for our café to grow with the needs and wants of our participating families and individuals, independently of any organizational philosophies and influence. To this day, we've remained independent of existing groups like the Alzheimer's Association and AARP, although we're most appreciative of their support and routinely refer caregiver guests to their support groups and programs. We work with a local non-profit group, which allows us to solicit tax-deductible contributions; but they do not participate in decision-making.

> "I sincerely agree with not being beholden to anyone. The hardest part I have found is keeping the cafe marketing free. There are plenty of places to sell your services, the cafe is a safe haven in all regards. I am also a Long-Term Care Ombudsman and this fits within protecting participants' rights.
>
> The director and another Ombudsman came to the last cafe for support and physical help. I have now added a VNA nurse too with whom I am working for Walpole's cafe. I love bringing everyone together and connecting people. Sharing resources is a positive experience for me."

Jean Cotton, MA

Formats and Programs

Many of the cafés in Europe offer counseling and presentations in addition to socializing. The Santa Fe eldercare community already offered several support groups as well as periodic workshops on Alzheimer's, dementia, and caregiving, so consequently we decided that our café would focus on the social and emotional needs of our guests. However, we always have experts on hand to offer support when needed.

Since we opened our doors in October 2008, we've had a steady crowd, who collectively decide our "programming." We have sing-alongs, make art, have discussions and always try to laugh a lot, all of it loosely planned. On Café days the back of my SUV is packed with assorted supplies for any and all eventualities: songbooks, art supplies, poetry and joke books, and of course, snacks.

"Consider a holistic approach: Think about how to engage a person physically, mentally, emotionally, and spiritually. This consideration should extend from the caregivers to those living with the disease. The more in-tune the environment, the more engaged and comfortable the attendees will be.

Include the Art. When you engage the arts, you touch the heart of a person. It's like giving them a hug without expectations, and that's definitely a spiritual experience. Music, dance, and crafts all fall into this category. Even if the person with dementia can't actively participate, they can still absorb the smiles, laughter and joy mixing around them."

Maryann Makekau, FL

Leadership

Leaders and volunteers don't need to be experts. Most important are an open heart and mind along with willingness to gain some understanding of Alzheimer's/dementia communication. Effective leaders of Alzheimer's Cafés come from all quarters. Many already work with programs for elders or people living with dementia and others simply have decided that this is something that needs to happen. In the case of our café in Santa Fe, my partners and I have years of experience working with the cognitively impaired and have no hesitation inviting people at all stages of dementia. Not everyone is ready for that, however. Since we're aiming for your success, I do think it's important that you are realistic about what you're prepared to handle. Some of the US cafés are directed toward a particular population, i.e., couples or people in the early stages only. In Santa Fe we have not found it necessary to screen or set any criteria for participation. Everyone is welcome, whether they have mild MCI or are in the advanced stages of Alzheimer's; or whether they are caregivers, family members or members of the community, simply interested in Alzheimer's.

Continuity and stability are important to your success, especially if you have an open door policy. In addition to a long-term commitment from your venue, you'll also want to bring in partners to help out and be ready to substitute for you when necessary. It's important that all of your leaders, including your volunteers have some understanding of how dementia affects people living with the disease and the issues typically faced by their caregivers.

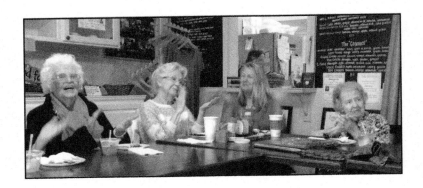

Naming Our Cafés

Our communities have come up with a variety of names for their projects. They are known variously as the Memory Lane Café, Forget Me Not Café, The Friday Coffee Club, and Neighborhood Café; Memory Care Café, J. Arthur Café, and Amy's Place. At a recent meeting of our Alzheimer's Café in Santa Fe, we agreed that there was something askew with using the word 'memory' for an event designed for people experiencing loss of memory. They compared a 'memory café' to holding a 'walking club' for paraplegics, someone suggested). Our group thought a more appropriate name would be the 'Confusion Café.'

Regardless of what we choose to call our cafés, they are part of a growing international movement, all having grown out of the original Alzheimer's Café in the Netherlands.

Why use a term as confrontational as *Alzheimer's* Café? Alzheimer's is the most prevalent of hundreds of cognitive disorders, representing between 65 and 85 percent of all dementia cases. There's a lot of misinformation about dementia in general and Alzheimer's in particular. This very word stirs fear in the public. As a consequence people living with Alzheimer's are especially at risk for alienation. Dr. Miesen started the Alzheimer's Café to provide a safe environment for everyone involved. He felt it's important to bring Alzheimer's into everyday conversations the way we have with other chronic conditions, like diabetes, scoliosis, or arthritis.

The first cafés in Britain were likewise known as Alzheimer Cafés, others since decided to use the name Memory Café, in some cases because some of their participants were living with different dementias, frontotemporal dementia (FTD), Lewy Body Dementia (LBD) or Parkinson's. More than half of the cafes in the US are known as Memory cafés.

Before you make your choice, you might take into consideration that we're part of an international movement and MEMORY is a word specific to the English language, whereas to non-English speakers, MEMORY may sound like gobbledygook.

These are the translations of "memory" in other tongues:
Albanian = **kujtim**, Danish = **hukommelse**, Maltese = **mœlu**

When the Alzheimer's Association started its annual fundraiser, 'Memory Walk', the term *memory* stood for commemorating someone who had died from Alzheimer's, not *memory* as in cognition.

"Many people living with dementia reject the term 'memory' cafe/walk/event/etc because it simply keeps the myth alive that dementia is only memory loss, which it is not. With some types of dementia, memory loss is hardly a feature.

In Australia, people have been setting up Memory Hubs, like a resource section about dementia in a library or pharmacy. I always suggest calling it a Brain Health Hub, as that's more useful and also supports people with other brain disorders, or who may be worrying about having dementia."

Kate Swaffer, AU

If you wish to acknowledge that your project is part of the international Alzheimer's or Memory Café movement, you might consider using Alzheimer's in the name of your café, as in "Henry's Alzheimer's Café." or indeed: "Confusion Club, an Alzheimer's Café." It will make it easier for people to find you in an online search. My online searches for a memory café in a particular locale usually provides me with lists of coffee shops named for flowers, birds, or lovely ladies, none of which is associated with dementia.

Getting the Word Out

Now that you have your name, your venue, and day and time, the next step is to get the word out to the community. I suggest contacting senior centers, churches, and home healthcare agencies, as well as support groups for caregivers. To get lists of support groups, contact the Alzheimer's Association, the Parkinson's Foundation, and Lewy Body Dementia Association.

Take advantage of social media, Facebook, Linked-in, Twitter, Instagram, and of course your own email contacts. Wherever you can, list your "opening" as an event, on Facebook for instance and local media calendar listings.

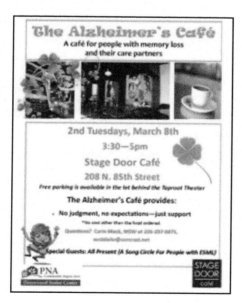

The Stage Door Cafe distributes monthly flyers

Contact your local TV and radio stations, online bulletin board, as well as your local newspapers.

And of course there's always the old-fashioned methods: snail-mail personal invitations and flyers and/or announcements. I create tiny handouts on print-yourself "business cards" and distribute to doctors, therapists, attorneys, trust officers, churches, senior centers, and any other place frequented by seniors.

One café leader suggest that we continue to remind support groups of times and locations of the cafes. Hilda Cook, who leads a memory café in Stamford Connecticut, says a quick phone call to members the night before their monthly get-together is appreciated and really helps boost attendance.

You're now part of a network of cafés. As soon as you're ready to start, we'll list you in the National Registry, Alzheimer's Café. You'll find that a lot of the leaders listed in the registry will gladly help you. We also invite you to join our Facebook group: Alzheimer's Café, to share ideas, post photos of your café, and connect with others. Many cafés start with a community celebration to set the right tone from the onset.

Chapter Four

What Happens at the Café?

Since we started the café in Santa Fe in 2008 we've explored all sorts of art projects, conversations, lighthearted joke sharing; sing-alongs, and music making. I routinely bring an assortment of art supplies, songbooks, joke books, and poetry.

The best cafés usually offer a combination of art projects or a physical activity, along with easy conversations, about our lives, childhoods, pets, and cookie recipes, often to find out that we have much more in common than enjoying being together at the café. At one particular café we discovered that all twelve of us at one point in our lives had lived or visited in the same small community in California. These casual chats appear to be much easier on our guests. When the pressure is off, the speech flows.

Not everyone is comfortable with a spontaneous go-with–the-flow approach. Some leaders prefer to work with themes for their programs, i.e., Valentine's Day, Summer Solstice, or Thanksgiving. Other cafés follow the 'European model' with a short formal session on dementia/Alzheimer's or specific caregiving issues, followed by a social or coffee hour.

"Thanks for the Memories, I brought a stranger and took home a loved one, for a while, memories for a time, even little memories are good, musical memories, laughing at oneself, he looked up and smiled, the marshmallows are on me! Small good times can be beautiful."

Frank Granberg, WI

One café in Erie, NY has been successful with a mix of activities that they do together, including memory games, crafts, exercise, and old trivia; Tai Chi, music, bean bag toss, have a golf tee, "What's in the Sock? Game," and Bingo (some cheating happens so the care partners win, not the volunteers.)

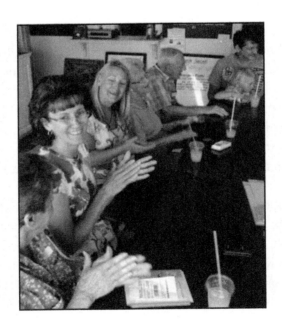

"We don't do the same things every month. Everyone loves the *Prize Basket,* filled with small donated items, some from health fairs, etc. Bingo winners often select a kid's item to take home to a grandchild.

It's important to be flexible and sensitive to the needs of the people attending. Some (care receivers) men just want to sit and talk. We have a retired judge and a professor who don't enjoy physical activities, but get into word games (with a volunteer discreetly joining in) and visiting with each other. Other men love the bean bag toss and get a rousing game going, including cheerleaders (usually the volunteers). Encouraging the women caregivers to do things with each other – they really appreciate the crafts – and we've seen them exchanging recipes and helpful tips. We always have a knowledgeable staff person present who can answer questions about dementia, services, etc."

Miriam Calahan, NY

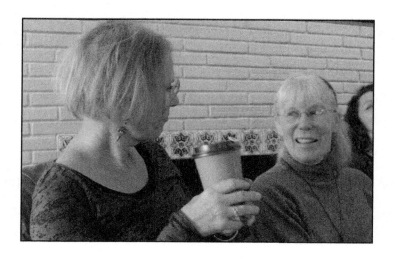

Comments from Café Leaders:

Q. What has worked particularly well for you?
Live music outdoors in the summer draws the best attendance.

Most enthusiastic response was to therapy dog visits.

Appointing one of the participant couples as communications directors and having them send out an email reminder every month.

Q. Problems you've had?
Attendance is erratic, sometimes 11, sometimes 2.

We're off to a slow start but it's picking up!

I wouldn't do anything differently.

Word is getting out and things are picking up.

Q. Anything else you'd like to add?
You don't need a lot of food. Our café is held at 2 pm; people tend to eat 1 cookie and have a drink and that's it.

For publicity, concentrate on word of mouth through agencies for the elderly and people with Alzheimer's.

Publicity efforts through ordinary media aren't very successful.

Need a group of committed participants for the first 6 months.

Remind support groups of times and locations of the cafes.

Opening Day in Santa Fe

As I was getting ready to opening the doors, I had searched high and low, but had not yet found anyone with experience in running an Alzheimer's Café in this country. I had no idea that our café would be the first one in the US, later confirmed later by fact-checking by AARP for a notice in the Bulletin.

I was a bundle of nerves as the day of my first meeting dawned. I had spent the last three months preparing for this, had hand delivered flyers to doctors, senior centers, and most of the churches and temples in town. Of course I arrived early, got everything set up and the sat in the room by myself for what seemed forever. I started fretting. I had prepared a generous spread of cookies, crackers, and nuts; chocolates, coffee, juice, and other goodies on the "buffet" – Was it going to be enough? – Had I given the musicians clear enough directions to find the venue? – What if this was a terrible idea? – What if nobody showed up? – Maybe I was doing all this in vain. – Maybe I should have paid more attention to all those colleagues who'd warned me that nobody would want to come to an "ALZHEIMER'S" café.

I need not have worried. It wasn't long before the room was alive with dozens of guests, chatting and laughing. Friends of mine had brought their effervescent marimba group to help us celebrate our grand opening. There was no question that people were having a great time. Half an hour into the festivities I noticed a lone woman leaning up against the wall, just inside the door. I invited her to join us, but she declined, firmly stating that she was waiting for "the Alzheimer's people" to show up – little did she know that about one-third of the crowd were people living with dementia. She could not distinguish one from the other. My instant thought was "What a sad example of the impact of the media." We've all seen the ads for Alzheimer's medications with actors portraying sad and depressed people.

Toward the end of our two hours, three women approached me. They told me that they were all in the early stages of Alzheimer's and were so glad to have found each other today. They loved the café and told me how thrilled they to have met others living with Alzheimer's. But could we please skip live entertainment because it was distracting and interfered with their getting-acquainted conversations?

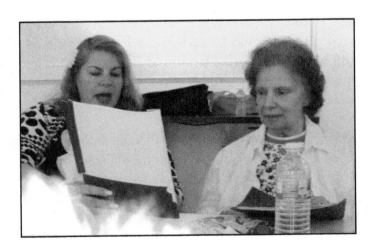

Chapter Five

No Two Cafés Alike

In this country, our cafés use a wide variety of approaches, some following the formal formats found in the UK and the Netherlands (*European model.*) The cafés in the Netherlands follow an agenda of presentations and discussions on topics of dementia and caregiving followed by a social hour.

In the United States we have as many different programs as we have individual communities. Most are centered on a social model with creative projects (*American model.*) The majority of the cafés in the US follow the *American model* and take into consideration the wishes and needs of their participants, so by their nature, our cafés are different one from the other.

A good example comes from the leader of two cafés in the same town who reports that both have programs according to the wants of the guests. At one café the group likes a very structured program with a short presentation and/or discussion on dementia and caregiving issues. On the other side of town, it's the opposite. That group simply wants to relax and have as much fun as possible with a variety projects.

All the cafés featured here are generously offering any of their ideas for you to adopt for your program.

Pasadena, CA

Right at Home in Pasadena made the decision to facilitate an Alzheimer's café to assist clients, their families and the extended community. Various Alzheimer's topic presenters are engaged to share the latest research, and offer various techniques and suggestions on how to better cope with and care for loved ones. This approach is known as the *European Model*.

"Sometimes it takes getting involved in your community to realize how prominent Alzheimer's is and how it is 'quietly' affecting many of our friends, family and neighbors.

At a presentation given by Susan Kohler, a licensed and certified speech-language pathologist, our members learned different methods to better communicate with their loved ones who are experiencing Alzheimer's. Members partnered up and ran through role-playing exercises that focused on key words, tips and redirecting attention to positive outcomes. Participation in the exercises allowed members to open up and ask questions relating to their particular situations. The members became familiar with each other, and learned they were not alone in their struggles. This was accomplished in a relaxed and friendly environment.

Our Alzheimer's café has grown in the last year through word of mouth and community outreach efforts by Right at Home. It is our hope at Right at Home, that we can provide a comfortable environment for those who are facing the challenge of Alzheimer's, to obtain information to assist them through this challenge, as well as give and receive support from one another."

Laura Koperski, CA

Seattle, WA

Half a dozen restaurants in the Seattle area have opened their doors to people living with dementia. Their Alzheimer's café events give families times to feel normal again with others, to laugh, sing, eat and "enjoy life the way they always used to be able to enjoy life," said one host.

The first café to open in Seattle was held in a very popular ice cream shop; it was soon followed up by half a dozen other cafés held in restaurants and pizza parlors. Restaurants like Tutta Bella in Columbia City provide customers a safe and comfortable place to visit. Several other local restaurants are now holding Alzheimer's cafés at no cost other than the meal. These restaurants typically provide a dedicated space and simplify their menus to provide customers comfort.

Dementia tends to socially isolate families. One husband said his wife would probably have stayed home in her pajamas had he not dressed her and convinced her to go out. "I comb her hair and put her earrings on her," he said.

At one cafe, a regular volunteer explains that patrons receive name tags. A guest says of his wife, "She'll recognize faces, but she just cannot remember names. The name tags help her feel comfortable."

Another participant, a minister and musician, had forgotten a lot of lyrics and chords due to his Alzheimer's. But his wife patiently guided him through his lapses as he entertained the group. Alzheimer's café has a very forgiving audience.

A welcoming atmosphere breaks down perceived barriers as it has done for one couple who's been married 56 years. "I'm not as sharp as I used to be," he says. "I think it's harder on my wife than it is on me." There's one thing his wife won't let him forget. "He's completely loved by God and by me and his family and friends," she says. "I want him to always remember that he's loved."

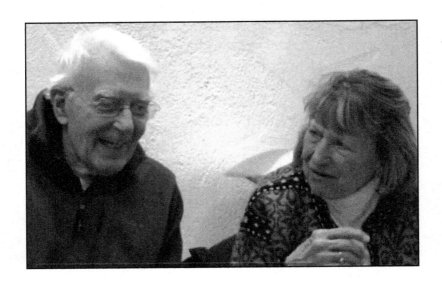

Marlborough, MA

Pleasantries is a successful home-based social model adult day program specializing in memory care for guests in the earlier stages of Alzheimer's or related dementia. Founded by Tammy Pozerycki in 2008, this unique program is located in a single-family home in a lakeside residential neighborhood offering the comforts of being at home or visiting a family member's home. Pleasantries provides full days of purposeful engaging activity for guests while providing relief and security for caregivers. When the director learned of the café movement, the closest café to her was in Dover, NH After attending it, she began the Create a Better Day Café on a Sunday afternoon at her Marlborough facility.

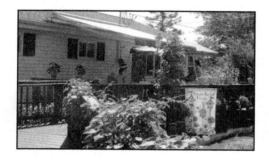

"It has gone from when I started with just myself and the food that I prepared – and no one else showed, – to now, when there are 15 to 20 guests with volunteers each month. We don't require RSVP. Someone who's caring for a loved one with dementia doesn't know until that exact day and time if it's a good idea to take them to a social event. Folks with dementia have good and bad days."

Tammy Pozerycki, MA

Roswell, GA

Amy's Place is a traditional home that has been remodeled to serve as a weekday program for elders. On the weekend, when it would otherwise sit empty, the community at large is invited to their memory café. This gives everyone an opportunity to share a relaxed and fun afternoon in a friendly and safe place.

"Amy's Place is a gathering place for those with dementia and their caregivers. We provide the opportunity for visitors to create new friendships. Amy's Place facilitates activities for the person with dementia. We host a variety of social events for families.

Support groups meet here. Amy's Place serves as a Community Resource Center for caregivers. Materials, tools, and resources are available through ongoing programming. We host educational events by accredited providers and volunteers.

We collaborate with local businesses that may provide resources and services to families. We provide community outreach to raise awareness about dementia and to reduce the stigma often associated with dementia and caregiving. Amy's Place creates a 'dementia friendly' community."

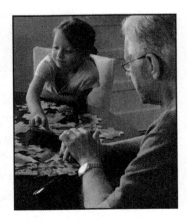

Pamela Jo Van Ahn, GA

Topsfield, MA

The Memory Café at REST. STOP. RANCH., MargFMac Front Garden Loop meets monthly during the months of April through October. Wheelchair-accessible, it offers a refreshing outdoor environment for care partners and individuals living with memory changes, at any stage of the disease process. Guests may enjoy music, dancing, laughter, conversation, and networking with people going through the same experience. Or they may choose to simply stroll through the beautiful gardens. The gardens offer a unique opportunity for quality time, memory-making, and idyllic photos.

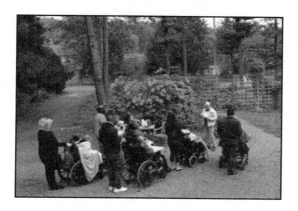

"What open-hearted, kind, generous spirits you are. You make me feel braver in this world knowing there are people like you out there. Thank you. When you tend to your garden, you are tending to so many tired hearts, but I think you know that already. You make this world a better place and we are grateful for it."

Patty and Steve, MA

The compact nature of the MargFMac Front Garden Loop accommodates the physical capacity and attention span of visitors. Guests of all abilities enjoy a rare opportunity to see and hear the birds, feed the fish, and get close to the plantings: see, smell, touch, pick and taste flowers and fruits. Multiple sitting areas provide spaces for contemplation and quiet conversations. The garden also offers areas for small group picnicking (carry-in, carry-out).

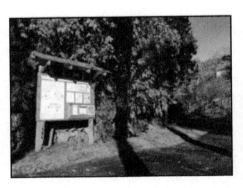

A street-side trailhead kiosk (built and installed, 2015) provides a way for neighbors to learn more about the Memory Café, leave a note, or sign-in as a visitor.

"It's weeks later and I'm still basking in the glow of sitting in your gardens. Just to sit on a bench! It was such a lovely respite for us. I find myself often revisiting that experience in my mind and in my heart.

What a gift to be able to enjoy such exquisite surroundings with the peace of mind that my Dad is safe, and is also enjoying Mary and Karl's home gardens. Their hard work at making the gardens accessible for persons in wheelchairs is so appreciated. My Dad and I are completely at peace and engulfed by the beauty of these gardens. The kindness shown to my Dad and to me, by Mary and Karl, is such necessary nourishment!"

Darcy Morales-Zullo, MA
(Pedro and Darcy drove over an hour to visit the garden.)

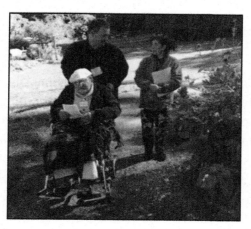

"After 10+ years of maintaining a life with early onset dementia, Joyce was more alert than I have seen her in very long time. Still now, three days after journeying over to your garden, the whole experience brings such tears of happiness to my eyes. To see my Mother-in-law so happy and so relaxed, is a wish come true!"

Lynne Marchetti, MA

Warner Robins, GA

The Café at Simply Cupcakes, is: "A happy, encouraging place. It is exclusively for people who are struggling with early to mid-stage memory loss, AND their spouse or care partner. It is a place of celebration and acceptance. It is place to look forward to visiting each month."

Every third Thursday of the month, the Café's programming features a different topic. For the month of June, they celebrated 'the good ol' summertime' and cut a chilled red Georgia watermelon, while reminiscing over a game of penny ante. For those not familiar with this card game, it is played in a round, with each person sharing their past accomplishments, feelings, and opinions, based on what question their card asks. We talked and laughed about everything from peanut butter to waking up early! It was a fun way to connect with each other, and learn how much we really had in common. Two people who had never met prior to the Café learned they once lived in the same small town.

July's theme: Travel. Guests are invited to bring a souvenir from a favorite vacation to reminisce!

Knoxville, TN

The memory café in Knoxville features dancing, singing, and indulging in delicious desserts and, according to participants, great company! Over their first four-year period they established traditions like an annual Luau in August, 1950s parties and "Thankful Feathers" projects in November. Typical of their events is a "Western Day" with everyone wearing cowboy hats and sheriff's stars, singing "Happy Trails" and Home on the Range" – as well as eating trail-mix and talking about their favorite westerns, movies, and stars.

At other times they have structured programs around simple activities, such as coloring a map of the US while talking about trips of old and trips they're dreaming of taking in the future.

> "When we did the map of the US, we heard so many stories about traveling around the country and around the world. We heard stories from elders that their family members had never heard. Our group that night was a very well-traveled bunch."
>
> Kathy Broggins, TN

Dover, NH

The second café to open in the country, the Children's Museum of New Hampshire has won the "Leaders In Innovation" award for the Alzheimer's Café program from the New England Museum Association.

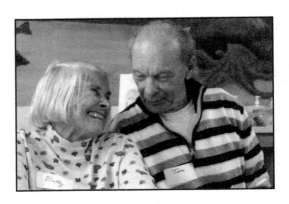

"We feel that our Museum is an ideal place for an Alzheimer's Café, We know that intergenerational experiences are beneficial for all ages, and we designed our Museum to be engaging for adults as well as children. Many elders did not have the experience of going to a children's museum as a child, so these visits give them the opportunity to see how we approach conceptual learning now, compared to what they might have experienced, and this always stimulates discussion.

The Alzheimer's Café program at the Children's Museum of New Hampshire in Dover was designed to address an unmet need in the community for people caring for a loved one with Alzheimer's disease or other dementias. Due to the unusual behaviors associated with the disease, people living with dementia, their families and care partners often face isolation, public judgment and criticism.

We noticed that Café attendees seem to enjoy themselves, and often form friendships that extend beyond the museum. Although Cafés are not for patient therapy, we observed they can have a beneficial affect, and that's what we wanted to study.

With the help of a nurse researcher and a graduate nursing student, a study was created using multiple methods of collecting data. In a published report, we share the results of the study, which highlights the benefits of coming to an Alzheimer's Café at the Children's Museum from the perspective of those who attend it."

Paula Rais, NH

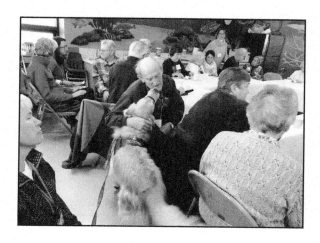

One man had been bringing his wife to the Alzheimer's Café in Dover, New Hampshire for several months. There he had connected with other husbands, who were also caregivers for their wives. As they got to know each other over the months, they realized that their issues were different from those of their female counterparts. They had different frustrations and different ways of coping with their daily tasks, many of which are not as routine for men as they would be for women, the cooking, house keeping, and alas . . . shopping for women's clothes.

As their friendship, these husbands started doing things together aside from the café and at one point collaborated on building a boat. Recognizing that they faced unique issues, they established their own men's support group.

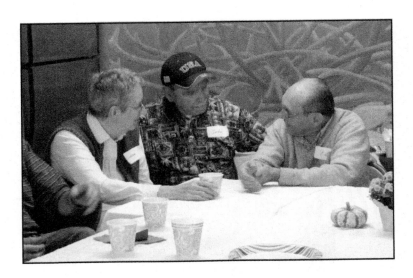

Fort Walton Beach and Destin, FL

Maryann Makekau sends out monthly invitations with brief descriptions of the events at the two cafés that she organizes.

"Engaging in a meaningful activity is like food for the soul. For individuals who have lost abilities due to dementia, the arts provide a chance to participate and succeed. The joy of taking part in a project, big or small, leaves a positive effect and contributes to a sense of happiness.

Activities have the added benefit of helping individuals maintain the dexterity and coordination needed to button a shirt, fold a towel or brush one's teeth, and more. Music fosters emotional connection and self-expression, and it has a way of bringing us back to a familiar time and place.

At the Neighborhood Memory Café we play up those interests and stimulate the inner artist – we've all got one tucked inside!"

Maryann Makekau, Destin, Florida

A typical calendar of the Neighborhood Memory Café:

September
Put on your blue suede shoes for some dancing music at the neighborhood memory café! On Thursday, September 24 at 3:00 PM come to the Synergy Organic Juice Bar and Café in

Fort Walton Beach for an incredible performance by Dan Mossman. He's a retired pilot who flew F-4s in the US Marine Corps. Then he spent 32 years as a commercial pilot before retiring from Delta Airlines. Dan now enjoys playing guitar and harmonica in The Mulligans Band and delighting crowds with impressions of Elvis (pictured here).

Then, on Wednesday, September 30 at Noon, come on over to The Breakfast Table Destin for a to-be-revealed surprise – and be sure to bring those dancing shoes again

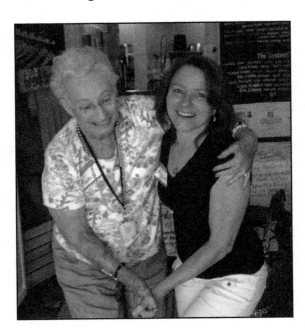

June

Did you grow up heading out to the lake on Sundays with Grandpa? Perhaps, you're among the 46 million Americans who fish today. Fishing is an activity that relieves pressure and creates a sense of fun and excitement. The sport is known to have a direct connection to health and well–being. We're going to capture those benefits at this month's memory café gatherings!

Join us for "Fishing for Tunes" - We'll literally fish for tunes in a pool of songs. You catch the tunes and we'll play the songs! Think of it like going to Disney to find Nemo!

April

Glen McClead will be joining us with his company of "Life Tunes" This month marks our 2-Year Anniversary at the Fort Walton Beach location. How time flies when you're having fun! A big shout-out to Synergy Organic Juice Bar and Café for hosting us and our sponsors and visitors - we couldn't do it without you!

We always like to close with a couple of shares to encourage you in this challenging journey. It's a fact, mental stimulation activities slow dementia. Every caregiver makes sacrifices to care for a loved one, whether it's putting aspirations on hold or rearranging priorities.

January

Terrie D. is going to visit us at The Breakfast Table in Destin. She is a Native Flute artist who brings a unique sound that easily engages listeners and inspires participation. Get ready for

Native Fusion, Jazz, Pop, Traditional, and Easy Listening of popular tunes through an array of instruments.

August

Meriel & Mercedes of The Full Circle Gallery will provide all the necessary elements to create pinch pot planters. You're guaranteed a refreshingly good time and an awesome take-home creation! The kitchen crew at Synergy Organic Juice Bar & Café will provide nutritious snacks to enjoy before we begin sculpting.

March

We're feeling eggstatic about the activities planned for next week's memory café! Easter is often referred to a season of renewal, and it's just around the corner. Immersing in the arts provides nourishment, whether listening to music or creating a masterpiece - it feeds our heart, mind and soul. So, we'll gather to create take-home works-of–art, celebrate caregiver milestones, create a nest egg (or two!) for the future, and love one another through it all.

Door prizes, delicious food and drinks, old and new friends await you at the Neighborhood Memory Café.

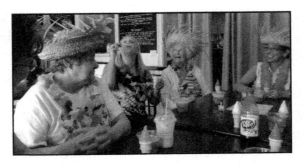

Fox River Valley, WI

The Fox River Valley was one of the first communities to promote the *dementia-friendly movement* and exciting programs throughout the area. This February calendar is typical of their calendars.

APPLETON. Appleton Public Library,
   Come to our tea (and coffee) party! We'll be talking about "all the loves of our lives" and will sing some great old-fashioned love songs. We'll also decorate some lovely heart-shaped cookies to donate to the Women's Shelter, with extras to bring home.

Atlas Coffee Mill and Café, 425 W. Water St. (In the Paper Discovery Center bldg) Thursday, Feb. 4, 2:00– 4:00 pm. Come and celebrate the LOVE dressed in Valentine Day colors. We will be led in song by Mary Schmidt of NewVoices. The musical theme of the day is LOVE SONGS. A "meet-up" to see the dress rehearsal of WEST SIDE STORY will be offered in lieu of the February, 18 Memory Café at Atlas.

KAUKAUNA: Kaukauna Public Library
   We'll take time to love ourselves for Valentine's Day! Barbara Fett, from Young Living Essential, will share information about essential oils and how to use them to enhance your mood and health. We'll also learn the art of relaxation and pamper ourselves a bit. Come and enjoy a nice break from the cold winter blues!

MENASHA: Menasha Senior Center

Join us as we "nourish the heart". We will share heartwarming stories and learn activities to keep our hearts happy. We'll also do an art project. Each month we are collecting recipes to make a recipe book at the end of the year.

NEENAH: Neenah Public Library

Join us for Tales & Travels from Africa. Pat & Jerry Rickman will take us on a trip to South Africa, Namibia, Botswana and Zambia. If you have traveled to Africa, please bring memories of your travels to share.

NEW LONDON: Mosquito Hill Nature Center

"Love Is In the Air"! We'll have a chance to hear about Greek mythology and love, reflected in the constellations we see each night. Join us to learn and create a special gift to take home. Music and refreshments will round out our afternoon. We hope you can be here! Feel free to drive up to the building to park.

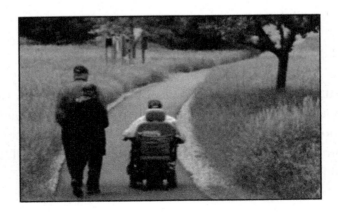

Brooklyn, NY

"We average 6 events per year. Our audience size ranges from around 30 people, up to 100 for one of our culminating events," says Gary Glazner, speaking of the Memory Arts Café. Gary is founder and Executive Director of the Alzheimer's Poetry Project.

"As a poet who has dedicated his life to working with people living with memory loss, I am primarily interested in creativity. All of the techniques I have developed with the Alzheimer's Poetry Project are participatory in nature and that holds true for the Memory Arts Café, founded in 2012. When I began planning how to structure our program the first thing I thought of was that I wanted to add the word 'arts,' to what are typically called Memory Café or Alzheimer's Café.

It was important to me that each event would feature a guest artist and that we create something with the artist depending on their genre, it could be a dance, song, story, poem or piece of visual art, or sometimes all these art forms at once!"

How we structure the Memory Arts Café:
"The first thirty minutes, we socialize over snacks and drinks and everyone has a chance to meet the guest artist. We take the role of host seriously and make sure people are getting introduced to each other and to the guest artist.

As the host of the event, I interview the guest artist for around 10 minutes. Not too long, but enough to get to know the person. I ask questions like how the person got started, a favorite or rewarding moment as an artist. I might ask them to explain a little of their art or if they are a musician talk about why they chose that instrument and how it works. The audience is encouraged to ask questions as well.

To end the interview section, I ask the artist to perform a short piece, around three to five minute long, so the audience gets a sense of their work. As a poet I often work with them and perform for example, a duet with dance and poetry or music and poetry.

During the next 15 minutes the guest artist creates a new work with the audience. A few examples of our guest artists include: Heidi Latsky, a choreographer who works with disabled communities and she created duets with us. The jazz singer Louise Rogers and pianist Mark Kross created a blues piece about Brooklyn. With visual artist Michele Brody we had a tea party! She brought in over-sized tea bags and fragrant containers of tea, which we smelled and then we wrote poem about tea on the bags as we sipped our tea.

Once we have created the new work we perform the piece with the audience. The key to the Memory Arts Café is that the performances are participatory. Everybody joins in and plays together.

We end the Memory Arts Café by again sharing food and drink, saying goodbye and socializing."

Gary Glazner, NY

"The Memory Arts Café lets us show participants how to communicate through the arts, through reading a poem, doing a dance, attending the Memory Arts Café. It makes it possible to meet people who are going through the same thing.

Support groups are wonderful but this is the ultimate support group. The families are communicating with each other and sharing the care, they are opening new doors on how to help each other. They are forming networks of support.

They are learning how to work with their loved ones better. Communicate with them better. Talk to each other about how they handle problems, without being stressed out so much. It's amazing. It's incredible the way they have come together. We have families that didn't know each other, but are coming to the Memory Arts Café and now they are going to each other's house for tea and planning BBQ's for the staff to thank the staff for bringing them together.

One caregiver has an appointment and can't get a home attendant and she has other caregivers to call and say, 'Can I drop my mom off and have you help with her.' It's paid back and they are sharing the care."

Josephine Brown, NY

Field Trips and Culminating Events

"While our home location is the New York Memory Center, we often take field trips and use the location to inspire the creation of poems, songs, and stories and our performances. We have had wonderful visits to among other locations, the Brooklyn Botanical Garden, Brooklyn Public Library, and New York Aquarium, located in Coney Island. In these locations we created poems about roses, books and jellyfish, respectively.

Once a year we hold a culminating event with a cultural partner and do out reach to the wider community to help build audience. We have had partnership with the Brooklyn Museum and performed at the Dweck Theater at the main branch of the Brooklyn Public Library."

Jellyfish

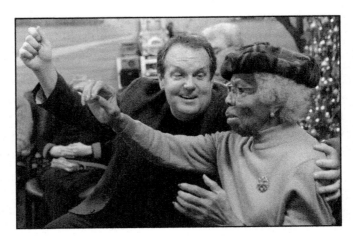

Photo: Michael Hagedorn

"People living with memory loss and their family members created this poem at the New York Aquarium in Coney Island on a field trip for the Memory Arts Café. We were inspired by the "Jellyfish-Alien Stingers," exhibit and created the poem by asking the participants to describe the jellyfish. We sang "Under the Boardwalk," and recited poems about the ocean including Walt Whitman's "The World Below the Brine," with its wonderful line, "... Different colors, pale gray and green, purple, white, and gold, the play of light through the water..." Poet Gary Glazner led the session. The Memory Arts Café is co-produced by the Alzheimer's Poetry Project and New York Memory Center."

Jelly, jelly, cha, cha, cha...
Jelly, jelly, cha, cha, cha...
They are just the cutest little things
I have ever seen.
Poooooofffftttt...
Stinging!
Strange!
Run for your life!
Run for your life!
Run for your life!

They are just the cutest little things
I have ever seen.

I hope they don't sting me.

Peanut butter and jellyfish!

A delicate balance.
A delicate dance.
A delicate balance.
A delicate dance.
Wearing our delicate jellyfish pants.

They are stingy and stringy and slimy.
They're fast.
They are beautiful.
Oh, I see a jellyfish.
How I wish they were on a dish,
Because I'm hungry!

They look like clouds floating in the water.
Tranquility.
Tranquility.
Tranquility and beyond.

Liquid buttons.
Liquid buttons.

Pooooofffftttttt…

How I wish they were on a dish,

Santa Fe, NM

The original Alzheimer's Café in Santa Fe, NM has been housed in the Santa Fe Children's Museum since 2009. Our guests love the colors, the cheerful atmosphere, and the energy of young children at play. Every so often a toddler will wander in to see what we're doing, usually when we're doing our best at our sing-alongs.

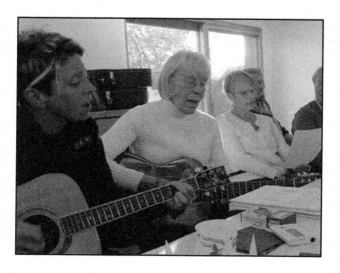

For the first several years at the Children's Museum, we had the use of the birthday party room, which had an official maximum occupancy of 16. Most of the time the space worked out just fine, but we did have a couple of large gatherings that stretched our space limitations. We were almost sitting in each other's laps. The room was appropriately festive, ready for a children's celebration. The drawback to the space was lack of running water (the closest faucet was a couple of rooms away) which put some limitations to our art activities.

After a couple of years, the museum underwent an expansion and remodel, giving us a new home in one of the classrooms, with running water and work tables, perfect for a wider variety of projects. It accommodates us comfortably, whether we're an intimate group of 4 or a lively party of 25. Should we need it, we can expand into the adjacent room. We have an open invitation to join the little ones at the Lego table, the water trough, the magic sound booth, or any of the dozen other fun activities.

"That day at the café has meant so much to me and my husband. I saw a part of him that I had not seen in a very long time. He was smiling, confident, uninhibited. These things have all been missing for the past seven years."

Deb Dalton, Los Alamos, NM

Chapter Six

"Dementia Friendly" Communities

An important mission of the café movement is the integration of elders back into the community on their own terms and simultaneously exposing the community to dementia. One indication that attitudes are shifting, is the evolution of programs for people living with cognitive impairment. Some communities have initiated "Dementia Friendly" movements in an effort to inform, prepare, and educate the public, making life easier for folks with various cognitive disabilities.

Several of my contacts who are living with dementia find the term "Dementia Friendly" disturbing. As one individual said, "I doubt we would accept the use of the term "Cancer Friendly" to promote equal and decent treatment of people living with cancer ?" Dr. Al Power suggest that we change it to "Dementia Inclusive" or simply "Inclusive Communities."

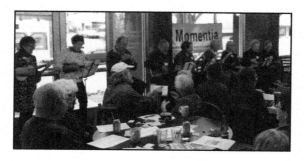

Momentia, WA

Momentia Seattle is one of the best examples of a program that's stimulating and fun, while promoting integration into the community.

Momentia Seattle celebrates *the new dementia story* as it spreads throughout the community, a story not of despair, but of hope and connection. The word **Momentia** is meant to be exclaimed as a cheer or rallying cry.

Momentia Seattle is part of a worldwide movement that's radically transforming what it means to live with dementia in a community.

As a movement spreading the new dementia story, **MOMENTIA** has three main components:

1. A joyful proclamation that people living with dementia can maintain full and meaningful lives in community, lives of creativity, connection, joy, purpose, health and strength. This story is told most vividly through the voices and experiences of people living with dementia.

2. An irrepressible community transformation with growing opportunities for people living with dementia to connect, engage and give back. The new dementia story is told through Alzheimer's Café experiences at neighborhood coffee shops, dementia-friendly art classes at local museums and parks, volunteer programs at the food bank, memory loss walks at the zoo, and more.

3. An irresistible invitation for everyone to work together, telling the new dementia story in creative and delightful ways: starting programs, creating films, talking with neighbors, writing articles, advocating for dementia-friendly improvements in your organizations, congregations and neighborhoods.

Momentia affirms:
- There is possibility for full and meaningful life with dementia
- People living with dementia remain a vital part of community and deserve opportunities to connect and engage as they always have.
- People living with dementia are the experts on their own experience and the authors of their own stories.
- People living with dementia demonstrate remarkable strengths and offer valuable gifts.
- A vibrant and healthy community is one that welcomes all its members to play a meaningful role.
- By working together, we can transform what it means to live with dementia in community, changing the story from one of despair to one of hope.
- Programs and events for people living with memory loss, their care partners, family and friends.
- Momentia is a movement transforming what it means to live with dementia, changing the story from one of fear, despair and isolation to one of hope, growth, purpose and connection.
- Momentia celebrates the courage and strengths of people living with dementia and creates innovative opportunities for engagement in and with community.
- Momentia is a story of living fully and boldly and finding joy in the moment.

- **Momentia programs:**

- Song Circle • Botanical Garden Walk • Drumming Circle •
- Gardening: In the Park and Urban Farm •
- Folk Dance • Art-Making Class and Gallery Tour •
- Improv Classes • Movies • Movement • Walking Tours •
- Food Bank • ESML Workshops • The Zoo and Aquarium

"The Momentia movement really speaks to me. I've been struggling with the wording, "Dementia Friendly," and how that was perceived. I wanted to take on a movement in Norwood, but Dementia Friendly did not resonate with me. Momentia Movement does.

I had been working with the Norfolk Adult Day Health Center on various things and always ask for input. The nurse said many of their clients missed going to the movies or theatre with their loved one. I asked the administrator of the Norwood Theatre if we could work something out for those, who want to attend, can and find a way to identify the shows. The woman said of course, right away! I could have movies at the cafe but why not have the normalcy and comfort of a public theatre. Everyone deserves that experience."

Jean Cotton, MA

Art Museums and Galleries

Memory loss from dementia rarely affects our other sensations and feelings. We may not remember what we had for breakfast, but we can still appreciate a beautiful flower garden or a colorful painting. Colors, music and art perception and appreciation linger even as memory fades. Our feelings don't diminish with memory loss, only the ability to express them.

Years before I'd heard of the Alzheimer's Café, I'd regularly take small groups of folks living with dementia on field trips. Depending on the season and everyone's wishes for the day, we'd go on picnics, scenic drives, and art galleries. Our hometown of Santa Fe, NM is considered the third largest art market in the US, so there's something for everyone. Depending on the mood of the day and the desires of the group, we might reminisce in a gallery of traditional realistic works or explore contemporary abstractions.

While we were out on these excursions, we'd collect images, pictures, and catalogs of the work we were looking at that day. Once we were back home, the pictures helped us when we'd talk about our experiences of the day and our thoughts about the art. Later these images would often be torn out and cut up to add to our collages.

Opening Doors

'Opening Doors' is an initiative that helps museums create programs that engage the senses and spark conversation for people with memory loss. No matter the size or collection, any museum or cultural center can create a customized tour to open the doors to the growing population of adults with memory loss and their families.

> "These tours are a powerful way to connect art with personal stories while engaging people with dementia in a life-giving experience. This pioneering museum work is a beacon for dealing with the age wave and consequences of dementia."
>
> Pat Samples, MN

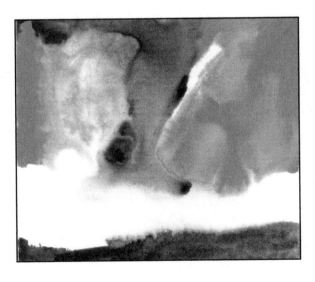

Museum of Modern Art (MoMA)

'Meet me at the Museum'
This appeared originally in ARTNEWS;
reprinted with express permission.

In 2011 the Museum of Modern Art (MoMA) in New York City pioneered a program for people living with Alzheimer's and their caregivers. Joan Mitchell's exuberant 1957 painting Ladybug prompted a lively discussion in a group of a dozen elders. [Non-figurative abstract expressionism, reminiscent of Jackson Pollack]

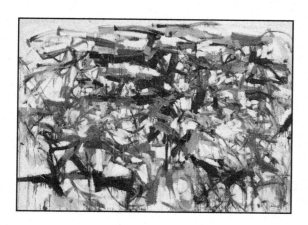

"It's chaotic," observed one visitor. "But it's beautiful chaos." Another member of the group suggested that it captured the spirit of spring. "No! It's set in winter," protested another. "Look at all that white." And a fourth participant offered up the ditty: "Ladybug, ladybug, fly away."

Had other visitors passed this group, they might not have guessed that the participants had something in common in addition to the their ages: Alzheimer's. Part of the museum's broader effort to reach diverse and underserved audiences-such as people with vision, hearing, physical, or developmental disabilities. The "Meet Me at MoMA" tours give people with dementia and their caregivers a chance to enjoy modern art.

MoMA's pioneering work with the Alzheimer's population began in 2006 with a pilot program at a nursing home, developed by Francesca Rosenberg, director of the education department's Community, Access, and School programs. In 2007, the MetLife Foundation awarded Rosenberg and her team a $450,000 grant to develop an arts–and–dementia program that could be adopted by other institutions. A second grant of $400,000 two years later funded an outreach effort that saw MoMA educators visiting institutions around the world to train museum professionals, caregivers, teachers, and health-care providers. A third MetLife gift, earlier this year, will underwrite yet more training.

In late March, more than 100 experts in Alzheimer's programming met at MoMA for a daylong summit. Museum educators from as close as the Metropolitan Museum of Art and as far away as Oslo and Tokyo gathered to hear neurologists, teachers, and Alzheimer's sufferers themselves discuss the disease and how an involvement with art can improve the quality of life for many patients and their caregivers.

Visual art is particularly well suited to helping Alzheimer's patients, research has found. According to Anne Basting, director of the Center on Age and Community at the University of Wisconsin, Milwaukee, art can trigger the emotional memory that often remains strong in Alzheimer's patients, and can give them access to other memories as well. And participants in art tours don't feel that they must already know something or that they will be expected to remember dates, names, or information. "The beautiful part of the program is that nobody mentions the word dementia. It's all about the art, and they can all connect to that. Nobody's sick, nobody's different," is how Kara Berringer, an art therapist at Pittsburgh's Carnegie Museum, explains the benefits of the program.

Research by the Ad Arte project in Naples, Italy, has demonstrated that exploring art encourages patients to speak and increases their self-esteem. Other studies have shown that people with Alzheimer's are able to rank their favorite colors, demonstrate esthetic preferences, and make associations between painted and real objects long after other kinds of memory recede. In St. Louis, the Pulitzer Foundation for the Arts builds on "profound ability" of Alzheimer's patients "to live in the moment" by bringing them together with schoolchildren who use storytelling and movement to enhance discussions about art. And, according to a recent report by the New York Consortium for Alzheimer's Research and Education, "there was a significant improvement in mood of both family caregivers and people with dementia that was measurable immediately, and sustained for at least a week" after art tours.

Diana Holbrook, a volunteer for "Meet me at MoMA," can attest to this benefit. Her husband, David, an original participant in the program, looked forward to the monthly outings. "I'm learning so much," he would tell his wife. They would talk all evening about the work they had seen that day. "For me, it was something I could enjoy with him. I didn't have to protect him," Holbrook says. After he died, in 2008, she became a volunteer.

A key component of the many programs seeded by MoMA and MetLife is that caretakers participate in the discussions, providing a fresh conversation about a shared experience and also helping to ameliorate the isolation of caretaking. As MoMA educator Riva Blumenfeld notes, "50 percent is for the caregivers rather than for the patients." She remembers a visit by an Alzheimer's patient and her curator daughter, who had an "amazing interaction" in the galleries. Being able to discuss art made the mother "proud of her daughter again, proud of what she did, and happy that they could connect," Blumenfeld said.

Institutions that offer Alzheimer's programming also stand to benefit. At the recent summit, Yale theater professor and critic Elinor Fuchs stressed that "engagement is the most important thing we can learn from this discussion. The learning process soars in groups." Fuchs is the author of a memoir about her mother's struggle with Alzheimer's, Making an Exit.

According to Amir Parsa, former director of MoMA's Alzheimer's Project (he is now chairperson of art and design education at Pratt Institute), working with Alzheimer's patients has changed education department pedagogy for all types of visitors. "In other educational interactions, we did not necessarily champion personal narratives intervening, because we were very focused on information transfer," he says. "With this group, we absolutely have to allow it. The digression allows them to internalize the meaning of the work in a very personal way. And we now believe we should allow this with all populations."

Back in the MoMA galleries for another tour, Rosenberg engaged her group in a discussion of Andy Warhol's Campbell's Soup Cans. One visitor said that she enjoyed looking for the differences and similarities among the cans. A second noted that the monumental series made her remember the different varieties of soup she ate in her youth. And a third observed that the paintings had greater impact as a group rather than as individual images.

Rosenberg described how a silk screen is made. She explained that the series represented each of the 32 soup varieties available when Warhol painted the piece, in 1962. "The label has been the same since the nineteenth century," she added. Then, describing Warhol's Factory and the social life his circle enjoyed at Studio 54, she playfully asked her group if anyone had ever been to either place.

Participants laughed and shook their heads. "And what were you doing in the '60s?" she asked. "Raising a family," responded one participant. "Working all the time," said another, shaking his head. Before returning to her script, Rosenberg let these memories linger for a few minutes, as her group smiled and reconnected to an earlier time.

Gail Gregg
Gail Gregg is an artist and
writer based in New York City.

Harlem, NY

Uptown from MoMA, The Studio Museum in Harlem offers the Arts and Minds Program, similar to 'Meet Me at MoMA' for less advantaged people who are living with dementia and their caregivers. After discussing the art, the participants get to create their own art in workshops.

> "Making art in hands-on workshops allows us to express ourselves creatively with or without words. Through shared aesthetic experiences, care partners learn that, despite cognitive changes, they are able to interact with a greater sense of who they are. Caregivers realize that there's still a lot to discover in their care partners."

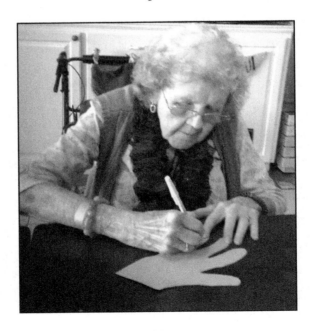

Taos, NM

ArtStreams combines immersion in art and creativity; social and personal support; educational resources; workshops and community collaboration.

One man reported that his wife, who had not spoken for a long while, went home after visiting an art gallery and began drawing again.

'Meet us at the Museum' brings family members, partners, friends and community members to selected Taos museums or galleries or in the Taos Fire Department Collections. We use art immersion as a tool to encourage observation, listening and sharing skills. The sessions are part story telling, part history and myth, and respite and social networking. Artists whose work we are discussing sometimes join the group with lectures and demonstrations of their techniques. Laughter is a big part of each session.

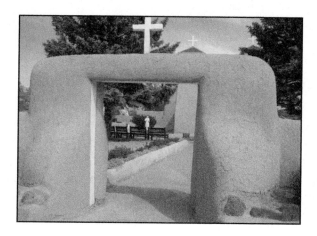

Albuquerque, NM

Like several other cafés, the Albuquerque café regularly invites their participants to bring their four-legged companions, much to the delight, emotional, and physical benefit of all the guests.

A few minutes of stroking a dog releases a number of hormones in humans, including serotonin, prolactin and oxytocin, all of which improve our feeling of wellbeing.

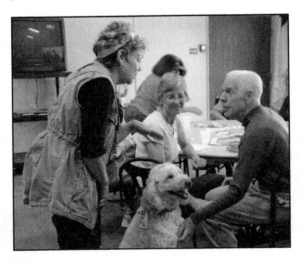

In addition, stroking a cat or dog decreases the levels of the primary stress hormone cortisol, the adrenal chemical responsible for regulating appetite and cravings for carbohydrates. Who knew that coming to a café is not only fun but also good for your health? Well, you might be as surprised as I was to learn that in 1859, Florence Nightingale promoted pet therapy for her chronically ill patients.

Chapter Seven

Music

In my workshops 'Memory is Overrated,' we focus on the parts of our brains that are not affected or only lightly affected by dementia, those parts that hold our perception and appreciation of the arts, including fine arts, dance/movement, and music. It's generally accepted that music is the very first sensation perceived at birth, possibly even in the womb, and is the last awareness to go at death. We may think that once our memories are fading, so is our ability to feel. This is not so. The memory and emotions aroused by music for instance pretty much stay intact. Often my friends, who had lost their ability to speak due to dementia, would join in a group sing-along of old favorites and not miss a word of the lyrics.

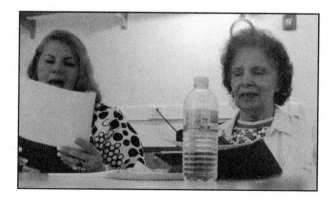

'Alive Inside' shows the power of music. This amazing movie documents a program initiated by social worker Dan Cohen to combat the isolation and loneliness experienced by residents in nursing homes.

Cohen had secured a grant to acquire hundreds of iPods. With the help of families, the iPods were loaded with music tracks known to be old favorites of individual residents. With the help of family members and nursing home staff, residents were introduced to the iPods with startling reactions. Seeing the residents listen to their favorite music choices is like witnessing an awakening. This movie is guaranteed to bring you hope and joy.

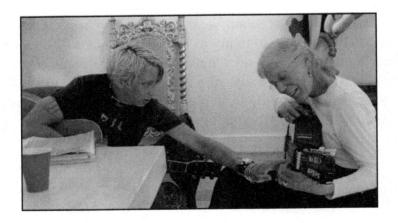

When we don't have a keyboard or guitar player around, we'll sing a cappella. Interestingly, the group tends to be more forceful in its participation without the accompaniment, maybe because we're free to choose our own pace and a register.

Over the years, we've been fortunate that some of our participants have been musicians. For several years one of regulars, who is living with Alzheimer's, would bring a beautiful guitar that she used to play decades earlier. Her companion and care partner was a musician in her own right, so the two of them would entertain us with their harmonies. We had the best time singing along with the John Denver and Beatles tunes.

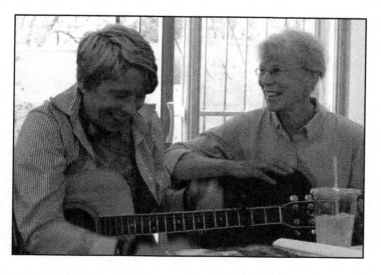

We weren't too bad, although at times our 'creative harmonies' (off-key) took over, giving us some good laughs.

"We'd invited a guitar player to accompany our sing-along. One of the regular caregivers has a good voice and loves to sing loudly. Her husband, an introvert, rarely talks and is sitting quietly, savoring his pizza. He has never joined in the singing. In fact, by looking at him you wouldn't know there is any singing. By the third song I coax his wife to join the guitar player at the front of the room. She joyfully begins selecting the songs and harmonizing in full voice. Her husband stops eating and turns to watch her. After a few minutes he stands and shuffles to her side. Slowly and deliberately puts his arm around her, smiles and looks at her tenderly. He stands by her so full of love and pride until the singing is over. His wife helps him back to his chair and he resumes eating his pizza in silence as if it never happened. My eyes fill with tears. What a beautiful moment. It validates our hopes for the café."

Melinda Franklin, WA

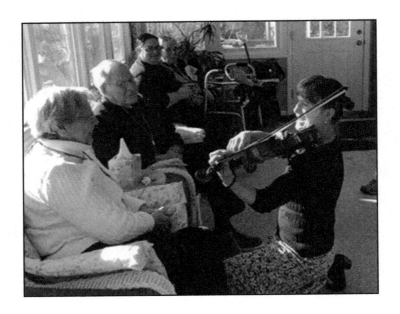

"At the very first cafe in Norwood, Massachusetts, the featured guest was Denis Galvin, director of Westwood School of Music. While he was playing his accordion, one of the guests was noticeably upset that other cafe participants were talking. Very loudly, she called out, "Stop!" The leaders asked the woman if she would like to sit close to Denis. She nodded her head yes. We helped her and her caregiver move right up next to the stage.

Denis heard the woman humming along with a tune he was playing. He paused after that song and asked her if there was a particular song she would like to hear. She said, "Danny Boy."

Much to the surprise and amazement of her caregiver, the woman started singing in a clear and confident voice. The microphone was passed to her and she accepted it right away. Everyone stopped talking and were solely focused on her singing. The caregiver began to cry and many at the cafe were taken in. Denis was also very touched. Now everyone was silent.

Her caregiver told us how she had loved to sing before being affected by dementia and how over the last few years, she had spoken very little and had stopped singing altogether.

We offered her a songbook to take home to sing to her family. She smiled from ear to ear. Everyone was touched by her performance and her caregiver's reaction. I was deeply affected by that experience and felt it had been an excellent validation of the importance of events like the Memory Cafe."

Jean Cotton, MA

Sing-alongs

When I first started our sing-alongs, I had inherited a stack of loose music sheets, copied out of various old songbooks, pages of 'oldies– but-goodies' mostly from the last century, i.e. 'Let Me Call You Sweetheart', 'Moonlight Bay,' and 'You are My Sunshine.' People started requesting more contemporary selections, so we decided to create our own songbook. We started by listing people's favorite singers and songs. Once we had a list that we all thought we knew well enough to sing a cappella, I'd print them and we'd try them out. Often the ones we thought for sure we knew gave us the best laughs, because we sounded like a pack of Siamese cats in heat. Many lively sessions later we'd have a new collection of favorites from the fifties and sixties, Frank Sinatra, Elvis Presley, Perry Como, and Patti Page's 'How Much Is That Doggie In The Window?'

We now have three regular songbooks, red, blue, and purple, plus the green holiday book, each with 20-plus pages, in large print. The books have different types of songs, giving us choices.

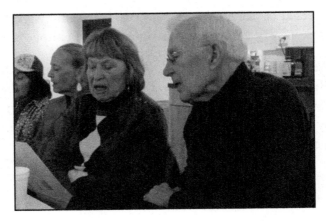

Starter Songbook

Sing-alongs are wonderful bonding tools, especially a cappella. One couple had come to a couple of our cafés when the wife said they probably wouldn't return because her husband had just been sitting there and didn't appear to get anything out of it. She then told me that he used to love to sing. I convinced her to try it one more time. The following month, as soon as everyone was seated, I asked him to choose which of our three songbooks we should use for that day. He sang with gusto and a big grin on his face. After that day, the two of them joined us regularly at the café. He not only sang with us but would also join in when we had projects, such as collages and tile painting. He also opened up and joined in our conversations.

I've included this short songbook to give you a head start,. You're welcome to copy these pages since they are in the public domain. Our more recent creations are songbooks strictly for private use, because of copyright issues. A couple of tips on creating your songbook: Use a large size font, minimum 18 pt. Number your pages, 22 pt in bold and limit to one song per page. I use three prong folders, which are usually inexpensive during back-to-school sales.

We recommend that you print one song per page in larger type (20-22 pt)

PAGE 1 – When The Saints Go Marching In

Oh when the Saints, oh when the Saints
Oh when the Saints go marching in.
I want to be in that number
When the saints go marching in.

Oh when the sun refuse to shine
Oh when the sun refuse to shine.
I want to be in that number
When the sun refuse to shine.

Oh when the Saints, oh when the Saints
Oh when the Saints go marching in.
I want to be in that number
When the saints go marching in.

PAGE 2 – Good Morning to You

Good Morning to You, Good Morning to You,
Good Morning to You, Everybody
Good Morning to You

PS This is a slightly revised version of the original "Good Morning to
You, Dear Children", which was composed in the early part of the
Twentieth Century by two sisters, both teachers of young children.

PAGE 3 – Shine on Harvest Moon

Shine on, shine on harvest moon,
Up in the sky.
I ain't had no loving since
January, February, June or July.

Snow time ain't no time to stay
Outdoors and spoon.
So shine on, shine on harvest moon
For me and my gal.

PAGE 4 – Give My Regards to Broadway

Give my regards to Broadway,
Remember me to Herald Square,
Tell all the gang at Forty-second Street
That I will soon be there.

Whisper of how I'm yearning
To mingle with the old time throng,
Give my regards to old Broadway
And say that I'll be there, e'er long.

PAGE 5 – Let Me Call You Sweetheart

Let me call you sweetheart, I'm in love with you.
Let me hear you whisper that you love me too.
Keep the love light glowing in your eyes so true.
Let me call you sweetheart, I'm in love with you.

PAGE 6 – Ain't She Sweet?

Ain't she sweet?
See her walking down the street.
Now I ask you very confidentially,
Ain't she sweet?

Ain't she nice?
Look her over once or twice.
Now I ask you very confidentially,
Ain't she nice?

Just cast an eye in her direction.
Oh me, oh my, ain't that perfection?

I repeat, don't you think it's kind of neat?
Now I ask you very confidentially
Ain't she sweet?

PAGE 7 – The Yankee Doodle Boy

I'm a Yankee Doodle Dandy,
A Yankee Doodle do or die,
A real life nephew of my Uncle Sam
Born on the Fourth of July.

I've got a Yankee Doodle sweetheart,
She's my Yankee Doodle joy.
Yankee Doodle came to London
Just to ride the ponies;
I am the Yankee Doodle boy.

PAGE 8 – Daisy Bell

Daisy, Daisy, give me your answer, do,
I'm half crazy all for the love of you.
It won't be a stylish marriage,
I can't afford a carriage,
But you'd look sweet upon the seat
Of a bicycle built for two.

Herman, Herman, Here is my answer true.
I'm not crazy for a man like you.
There won't be no kind of marriage
You can't afford a carriage
And I'll be damned If I'll get crammed
On a bicycle built for two!

PAGE 9 – Moonlight Bay

We were sailing along on moonlight bay.
We could hear the voices ringing,
They seemed to say:
You have stolen my heart, don't go away.
As we sang love's old sweet song on moonlight bay.

We were sailing along on moonlight bay.
We could hear the voices ringing,
They seemed to say:
You have stolen my heart, don't go away.
As we sang love's old sweet song on moonlight bay.

PAGE 10 – Take Me Out to the Ball Game

Take me out to the ball game,
Take me out with the crowd,
Buy me some peanuts and Crackerjacks,
I don't care if I never get back.
Let me root, root, root for the home team
If they don't win it's a shame
For it's "one, two, three strikes you're out!"
At the old ball game.

Dancing – Movement

My portable CD player comes in handy for our impromptu improvisational "dances." Some of us are not too mobile so we've come up with some interesting moves, such as variations of 'chair dancing.' We're not really concerned if Arthur Murray wouldn't have approved, because we have some great laughs and our bodies get a bit of exercise.

One of our guests, who was in a wheelchair, got everyone engaged in a chair ballet to the 'Humming Chorus' from Madame Butterfly. We quickly went from feeling silly to being mesmerized.

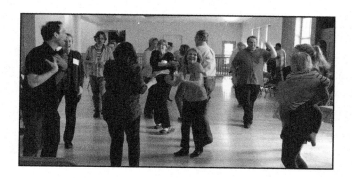

Art and Dance Event

Gary Glazner shares his talents with communities in the US and around the world. He collaborates with local museums for his appropriately named 'Community in Residence' programs. One example is an event held a the New Mexico History Museum: A collaboration with Maria Genné from Kairos Dance Theatre of Minneapolis, who lead a couple of hours of invigorating and fun (but easy) dance routines. Backed by uplifting music in a clear beat, we started out just walking to the beat in a circle, then in a twisted circle and at some point everyone started going into their own solos. At times the laughter almost overwhelmed the music. It was so simple and yet great exercise and joy.

Word Games

Gary Glazner has brought his unique approach to poetry into the Alzheimer's community. Just like old songs awaken people locked into their dementia, classic poetry can do the same. Gary will recite a short verse from a familiar poem, starting in a normal tone and then repeating the verse, building up to exaggerated vocalizations and gestures.

By the third or fourth repetition the crowd is fully engaged and participating, gesturing and laughing. The point is not the poetry per se, but rather the feeling of familiarity and being in a happy and noisy group experience. Imagine how powerful this can be for a person who's generally locked in his own world. Especially if he's living in an environment that tends to be low-key with little overt expression of joy.

After this introduction through a shared experience, Gary often engages the group in creating their own poetry. He may use a painting as an inspiration, calling on individuals for words to express their feelings and thoughts about aspects of the painting.

An assistant writes down everything said. After an energetic give and take for around ten minutes, Gary will lead a call–

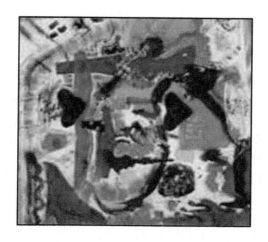

and–respond reading of the list as a free form poem. His secret is that he infuses his reading with the same exuberance, animation, and gusto that he uses when leading the recital of traditional poetry.

Drama – Theater

I love Gary's approach to poetry; it's such a natural lead-in to goofy role playing and loosening up with a bit of nonsense. You don't have to use actual poetry, a verse of an old standard tune will do just as well, i.e. 'Let Me Call You Sweetheart' or 'Mary had a little lamb.' It really doesn't matter; it's all about the energy we put into our renditions.

The 'Happy Times Café' in Sacramento combines word games and drama. Using a painting, the group wrote down what they saw in the image. People saw hockey games, music, and young lovers. They followed up with a make-believe session of being in a TV drama, making up the storyline and playing the different characters. They managed to write down their creation, before everyone dissolved into laughter.

We have also had fun with recreated some of our favorite scenes and characters from theater or film that are familiar to pretty much everyone. Judy Garland's 'Toto, I don't think we're in Kansas anymore.' Brando's 'Stella! Stella!' or Marilyn Monroe 'Happy Birthday, Mr. President,' Clark Gable 'Frankly my dear, I don't give a damn,' Lauren Bacall, 'You know how to whistle, don't you? Just put your lips together and blow.'

It is so rare that we grown-ups have a chance to act goofy. The café give us a chance to let down our hair and forget about appearances. Since there is no requirement to remember anything, all these engagements are for pure, unadulterated pleasure.

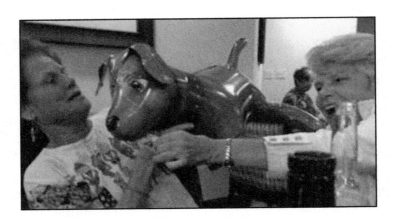

Fun and Laughter

As you have probably noticed, one very important component of all these exercises is laughter. Laughter is incredibly powerful. Laughter improves our heart health, our blood pressure, and circulation. It strengthens the immune system, reduces stress, and increases the endorphins and dopamine in the brain, leading to a feeling of wellbeing.

Most importantly laughter has no language barriers and is an instant bridge between humans. Connecting with others and socializing are as important to us as a healthy diet. Along with a song or two, laughter creates a feeling of kinship in the group. It's natural to follow up with warm hugs.

We always make sure to include laughter at our café. Although we've hardly ever needed it, I keep a ring binder of funnies with me at all times, to make sure that each café always offers a healthy dose of giggles or guffaws.

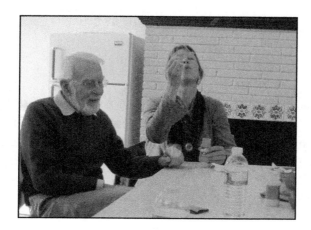

If funny stories or jokes don't do the trick, you can always try 'laughter yoga' – Laughter is so irresistibly contagious that soon the group will follow.

At a Fox Valley Memory Café in Appleton Wisconsin, facilitators John and Susan McFadden reserve time near the beginning of their café for people to share jokes. Susan says, "After welcoming everybody, we often have what we call 'Bad Joke Time' where people bring in their worst jokes. This is VERY popular!"

The single all-time favorite joke of all my groups over the last twenty-plus years:

> Jack meets Joe on the street. Jack says,
> "Hey Joe, you gotta get blinds for your house. I drove by your house last night at nine o'clock and I could look right into your living and I saw you making love to your wife right there in your living room."
>
> Joe slaps his knees and laughs as he says,
> "Hahaha, the laugh's on you!
> - - - I wasn't even home last night"

I also maintain two fat and growing ring-binders, one of 'Stupid Laws,' actual laws that are presently still on the books, the reasoning being that they are so unreal that they'd be thrown out of court immediately.

Example: • *It's illegal to shower naked in Florida.*

Chapter Eight

Creativity

'Activity programs' offered by care facilities are typically passive. Residents are entertained rather than challenged intellectually or creatively. I collect activity schedules from around the country. The typical schedule offers activities in one-hour slots, similar to class schedules. In most cases, residents are offered at most two one-hour sessions a week of arts or crafts. I have yet to meet a professional artist who is able to do much creating within an hour. Every one of us has our personal internal clocks that dictate how long it takes us to process new information or recall old knowledge. People with cognitive deficits typically need extra time to focus on any project, whether it's old or new.

As a teacher I had considerable success with programs that allowed students the time, tools, and space they needed to work at their own pace. When I first introduced projects into a dementia care community, I instinctively followed the same philosophy and found that my approaches worked equally well with teen-agers and people living with dementia. The secret to our success was time and choice. Everyone responds to something that gives her a purpose. It can be something as simple as filling a folder with cutouts of horses, experimenting with laying out strands of beads in designs, or crocheting baby bonnets for newborns at the local maternity ward, all of which were real projects of some of our participants.

The projects presented here have all been tested and approved by our café. They are doable within our time constraints, which for most of café is two hours.

There's no right or wrong

A poem does not have to rhyme.

A sing-along does not have to be in key; (We call it creative harmony)

A painting or drawing doesn't have to look like something

We can dance to our own rhythm

Making Art

Dementia affects people's memory, speech and may also affect comprehension, but remarkably other parts of the brain appear to function normally into the more advanced stages of the disease. Music awareness and enjoyment appear to linger to the end of life. Emotional reactions to color and artistic expression also last long beyond the memory loss, as does a person's ability to create. My groups had been busy painting, drawing, and making collages for a couple of years by the time I was told by a few "experts" that people with dementia lose the ability to learn new skills. I was too new to the field to contradict them, after all, I had only worked with a couple of dozen people for two years at the time. However, several members of my groups had gotten very skillful with tools and materials.

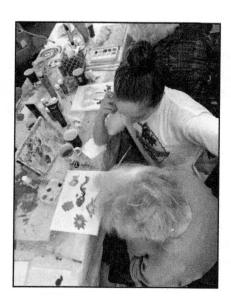

Collages

When I first suggest art projects to adults, I inevitably run into a wall of protests. "I have not talent." "Oh, no, I wouldn't know where to begin." "I can't draw, or paint, or whatever"

It's hard to convince people to go ahead and give it a try, even when we remind them that there's no right or wrong. Whenever we contemplate creating something, most of us will automatically start to formulate images in our minds, images most often beyond our capabilities, so we're setting ourselves up for failure. By the way, most professional artists do the same thing, except we understand that these imagined masterpieces are simply inspirations.

Rather than force the issue, I'll start with a group project, which I've found is the most effective to ease folks into the creative process, usually a large collage. When you have several people working on the same collage, even with the smallest effort, everyone automatically has ownership. So it doesn't matter if you've contributed six intricate cut-outs or one tiny sliver. The group project automatically eliminates competition.

One of the most powerful experiences with a group collage happened in a care facility. Albert was in the late stages of Alzheimer's and Parkinson's; his speech was limited to a few single words, mostly juicy profanities. Daily I would offer to roll his wheelchair up to our creative sessions. He would typically dismiss me with a swipe of his hand. Instead he spent a lot of time shouting at us from the other end of the room. This lasted a couple of weeks before curiosity won out and he allowed me to wheel him over to join the group. He gestured toward the scissors and paper, but refused my offer of assistance and spent the next hour cutting a tiny red sliver, a painstaking process due to Parkinson's and his trembling hands.

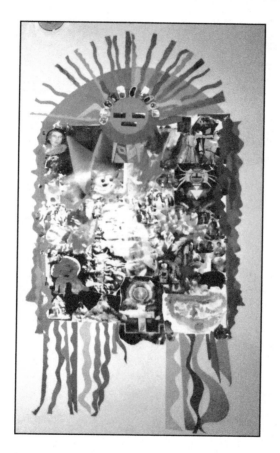

If you look closely at the collage above, you'll see Albert's little red sliver at bottom right.

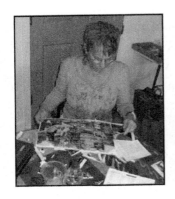
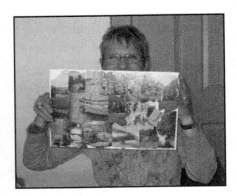

It probably won't take long before participants will want to create their own. We use mostly art magazines for collages. 'Making art from art.'

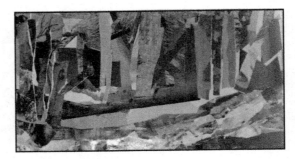

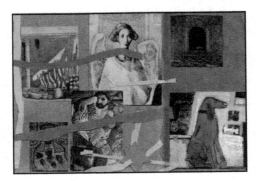

Group Painting Project

If you have a space that can accommodate it, a large group painting can be another spectacular project. This is from one of Gary Glazner's community events. We covered the floor with painters' drop cloths over butcher paper.

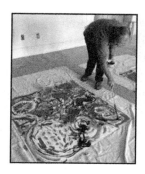 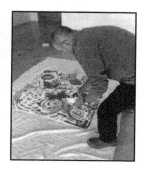

Gessoed 4' x 4' masonite boards served as "canvasses." We used inexpensive poster paints, foam brushes, sponges, twigs, hand brooms, sticks, and very long handled paint brushes. We also added texture with crumbled tissue paper and a little bit of glitter, attached with ModPodge. Six to eight people participated in this project

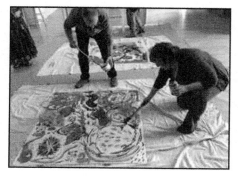

Painted Tiles

Tile painting is the ultimate no-fail project and remains the most popular of all our creative endeavors at the café. It requires an initial investment in supplies, but other than that, it's a simple project to set up and it's easy to guide novices in the few simple steps.

One person in particular impressed all of us. Elsie was living with Alzheimer's and the effects had advanced to the point where she was no longer able to participate in most of our group fun. Most of the time she was grumpy and would have loud, often profane, outbursts. This had gone on for months, until the day I brought in a stack of white tiles and special tile paints. She quieted, watched with fascination and picked up the tools. From then on, Elsie would greet me with a firm declaration: "Tiles!, Tiles!" and would cheerfully paint tiles at every single session. She painted more tiles than everyone else. It's especially remarkable that she learned to control all aspects of the craft and was very deliberate in her designs. She proved the specialists wrong.

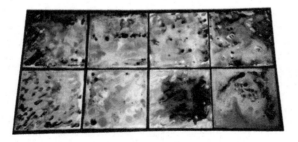

Elsie never learned my name (it *is* pretty tricky) but she certainly knew who I was.

Tiles How To

Tools and Materials:
- Porcelain or ceramic tiles (we use 4" white tiles)
- Porcelaine® brand paint. We tested several similar porcelain and glass paints and found this product superior to the rest
- Q-Tips

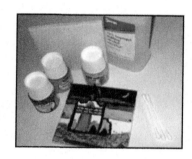

Optional:
- Denatured alcohol
- Plastic cup
- Eyedropper

How-to:

Cover your table with a plastic tablecloth.

Choose 2-3 colors – more colors easily turn to mud

Scoop a small amount (pea–sized) of Porcelaine® onto a small disposable plate

Pour a small amount of alcohol into the plastic cup

Clean the tile, plate, or cup with alcohol.

Wet your Q-Tip with alcohol

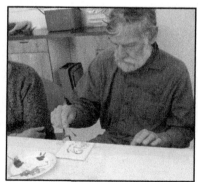

1. Use one Q-tip per color and give people extra Q-tips to use for mixing.

Apply a dab of color into a "puddle" of alcohol on the tile. If it doesn't start to flow, drip a little more alcohol over it. This is where an eye dropper comes in handy. You can also use a make-up sponge or a small foam brush; either will allow you to squeeze out a small amount of alcohol. If you're doing this project with a resident, you may have to 'assist' by doing the alcohol sprinkling.

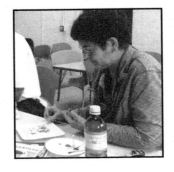

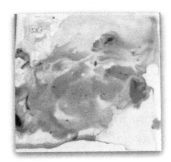

Recommendations: An experienced person "controls" doling out the paints in small dabs.

Note: Of course you don't have to use this particular method. You can skip the alcohol and use the Q-Tips in place of paint brushes.

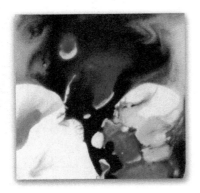

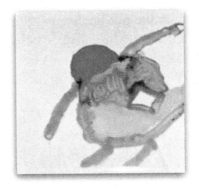

120

Holidays and Celebrations

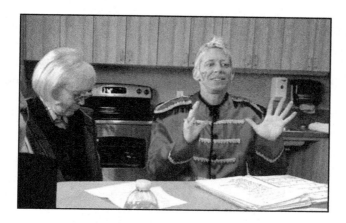

Valentine's Day

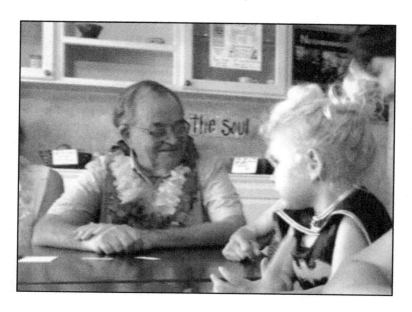

Easter: Decorating eggs:
1. Boil eggs in water with food coloring or crumbled colored tissue paper.
2. Draw design on hardboiled egg with crayon or a white utility candle before dipping in lukewarm water with food coloring.

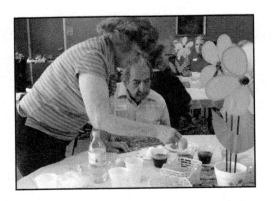

3. For eggs not meant for consumption you can decorate the surface with yarn, stickers, glitter, skinny ribbons, or magazine cut-outs

Halloween

Instead of carving pumpkins, you can draw on them with permanent markers, glue on glitter stars, cutouts, feathers, or you can dress them in flowing tissue "gowns"

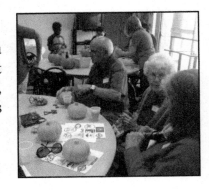

The Happy Times CAFÉ in Sacramento mounted an art show in collaboration with local assisted living facilities.

Some cafés have had success with creating arts and crafts for fundraising for their cafés and other organizations.

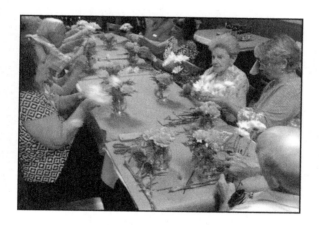

Poetry and Story Writing

Stuart Hall was a prolific poet, or as he preferred to call himself a 'versifier.' He made the best of living with an undetermined dementia by writing constantly. We were privileged to have him as one of our regulars at the Alzheimer's Cafe. The New Mexico History Museum is publishing a collection of his work.

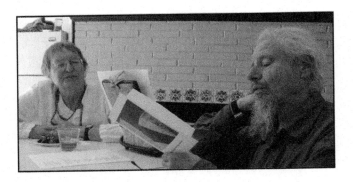

North Wind

How tightly rose-petals adhere!
You'd certainly think that the mere
    Hint of this wind
    Would make them rescind
Any claim they might stake to stay here.

The common red-eyed Drosophila
's as acute as your average philosopha,
    Who (you'll find) to the core
    Is a terrible bore
At the least; or even awfulla
['Drosophila' is a genus of small flies, often called fruit flies.]

Chapter Nine

Alzheimer's and Related Dementia Basics*

"Dementia" is not a disease as such, but rather an umbrella term for symptoms common to hundreds of different brain disorders. Frequently known as senility, dementia is commonly associated with Alzheimer's disease, but is often mimicked by other old-age problems such as depression or overmedication. Dementia symptoms include a progressive loss of cognitive function, problem-solving abilities, remembering, attention span, and language skills. Early signs are memory problems and confused thinking. Dementia is on the list of *neurological disorders.*

*The following is a synopsis meant only as a brief overview. Go to ADEAR.gov or Alz.org for details.

Alzheimer's Disease – accounts for sixty to eighty percent of all dementia cases. This type of dementia affects memory, especially short-term memory, problem-solving, attention span and language skills.

Vascular Dementia – accounts for another 10% of dementia cases. The first signs of vascular and multi-infarct dementia are impaired judgment, inability to make decisions, plan or organize, and increasing difficulties with money matters.

Balancing the checkbook, forgetting to pay bills and being vulnerable to con or scam artists is more likely to be the initial symptom, as opposed to the memory loss often associated with the initial symptoms of Alzheimer's.

Mixed Dementia – Alzheimer's combined with another type of dementia.

Lewy Bodies Dementia – Similar to Alzheimer's. Prone to hallucinations.

Frontotemporal Dementia – Damage to the front and side regions of the brain. FTD causes difficulties in thinking and behaviors controlled by the frontal and temporal parts of the brain. Symptoms can include strange behaviors, lack of empathy and foresight; emotional problems, trouble communicating, or difficulty with walking and other basic movements.

Parkinson's Disease – Many people with Parkinson's disease also develop dementia.

Pick's Disease – A type of frontotemporal dementia.
Other causes of dementia include Huntington's disease, Creutzfeldt-Jakob disease, head injury, and HIV.

Alzheimer's is always dementia,
but dementia is not always Alzheimer's

Warning Signs:

At some point we have all forgotten something: where we put our keys, the names of people we met last week, the container of Chinese takeout from last month that's now a "science experiment" sitting in the back of the refrigerator, or to pay a bill. However, when a person shows several signs consistently, it's time to become proactive. In addition to memory loss, other signs are changes in behavior along with a decline in cognitive ability and often personality changes. Also hoarding behaviors, stashing common items in strange places i.e. toothbrush in freezer or ice cream in closet. Forgetting personal care routines, i.e. eating, bathing, or changing clothes. Increased anxiety, suspicions, and accusations.

TEN WARNING SIGNS

1. Memory loss that disrupts daily life
2. Challenges in planning or solving problems
3. Difficulty completing familiar tasks at home, at work or at leisure
4. Confusion with time or place
5. Trouble understanding visual images and spatial relationships
6. New problems with words in speaking or writing
7. Misplacing things and losing the ability to retrace steps
8. Decreased or poor judgment
9. Withdrawal from work or social activities
10. Changes in mood and personality

Remember: There's much more to each of us than our memory and even when our personalities change, our personhood stays intact until our last breath. Keep in mind that no two of us are identical and this is especially true of people with dementia and Alzheimer's.

Reversible Dementia and Delirium

Before you assume that a loved one has dementia of one of the incurable types, you'll want to eliminate possible reversible causes, such as normal pressure hydrocephalus, thyroid problems, and vitamin B deficiency, can be reversed with appropriate treatment.

Normal Pressure Hydrocephalus (NPH) – Brought about by the buildup of cerebrospinal fluid in the brain. Causes problems with thinking and reasoning, walking and bladder control. If diagnosed early, it can be relieved by the insertion of a shunt.

Other reversible conditions that mimic dementia:
Drug reactions, malnutrition, dehydration, and vitamin deficiencies; infections, anesthesia, and illnesses. Depression is by far the most common of the potentially reversible conditions. At the first sign of acute confusion and memory loss, see your doctor; a sudden onset of confusion or delirium may indicate a reversible condition.

Words Matter

The words we use affect our feelings toward our situations and the people in our care. If we talk and think of caregiving as a burden, it most certainly will be so. When we call a person an empty shell, we'll think of her and treat her as such and she'll likely withdraw into herself and "prove" us correct.

We don't normally identify people by their disorders or diseases: i.e. If we have chronic conditions like diabetes or scoliosis, we wouldn't want to be referred to as a diabetes person or scoliosis person, would we? How would feel if these words were used about you?

Alzheimer's person, demented person should be "A person living with Alzheimer's or dementia"

Crippling, Demented, Victim, or Sufferer; Invisible, Fading, Not all there, Empty shell, or Losing it. These terms assume that we should use our own standards to judge others. Well, in that case, whose standards? – yours or mine?

Behavior problem, challenging behaviors, and difficult behaviors. Often the "problem" is with the caregiver and a lack of understanding communication. A person who has lost his ability to communicate with words will resort to other ways. If he's frustrated that you don't get the urgency of his problem, he may flail, gesture, make loud noises or even strike out. We call this "behavioral expression." – What would we do if we were stuck in a foreign country and needed help but didn't know the language?

Vocalizer, Aggressor, Wanderer, Sundowner, or Feeder. We don't describe each other by our actions, so why do so with people with dementia? We have stripped them of their humanness.

Fighting Alzheimer's, War on Alzheimer's, Win over or beat Alzheimer's, or Battling Alzheimer's. Combative terms keep us in a negative and often hopeless state. Until we come up with a cure, Alzheimer's and other dementias are chronic conditions and for everyone's sake, let's make the best of our situations.

The term *Patient* is relevant only in a medical sense. Doctors, nurses, dentists, therapists etc have patient. The rest of us have residents, clients, friends, etc.

Memory Care and *Memory Café* are oxymorons that may be offensive to people with dementia. We understand that it would be inappropriate to announce a "walking" club for paraplegics.

And lastly *The Long Goodbye.* Pleeeeeeease!!! This may be the most cruel of all. Does this mean that a person starts dying as soon as he is diagnosed? The truth is we're all dying a little every day of our lives. So, to borrow from Dr. Richard Taylor who lived well for over ten years with a diagnosis of dementia, probably of the Alzheimer's type: "I'm still ME, so let's say HELLO"

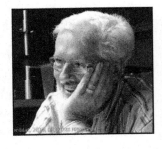

The biggest change for me since having dementia, is that my language was beginning to diminish so much that I found myself not talking, preferring instead being silent. When people asked me a question, I could not get the words out or I could not remember how to speak. Taking up pottery has changed my life. I have something that I love to do. Now after 2 years, my language expression is better, not totally back, and there are still many moments when I am in what I call la la land when someone is talking to me. Yet, more often, I can carry a conversation for a while before anyone could tell that something is not quite right; that I'm struggling for the words or not being able to remember what something. My ability to speak, being able to form words, and speak them clearly has begun to improve."

Susan Balkman, NM

Communication

Regardless of the cause or causes of the dementia, appropriate communication is crucial to avoid further stress and aggravation. These are the basics of effective communication:

Listen!

Avoid Baby Talk — use normal adult speech

USE COMPLIMENTS AND HUMOR (a lot, — but never at your companion's expense)

NEVER ARGUE OR ADMONISH

Avoid: "Do you remember?" ...

Avoid using the word: *NO!*

Use Diversions and Appropriate Reactions

Respect altered realities*
I use this term for when a person with short-and mid-term memory loss goes back to relive a situation from childhood.

Chapter Ten

Surveys

Over the years we've had discussions on how to gauge the success of our cafés. We had all been witnessing the positive changes in individuals and relationships, but how do you measure happiness?

Our first informal survey was in 2013 we reached out to the cafés at the time. Since then the cafés in Dover, NH and Boston, MA, conducted formal surveys.

2013 Feedback

• What has worked particularly well?

Asheville, NC: I felt the need for the Memory Café because I run support groups for people who have a diagnosis and it was clear that they were all hungry for social activities for more interaction together in between our support group sessions. It also became clear that the couples (caregiver and person with diagnosis) needed to have something they could both enjoy.

The casual drop-in nature of the Café makes it easy for people to test them out, stay as long as they want. We have been fortunate to have many couples attend several of the café, giving them 4 locations over the course of a month for a social activity together. Live music at various Café events has been a big hit – we've had hammer dulcimer, guitar, piano, and sing-alongs.

Brooklyn, NY: For our one year anniversary we partnered with the Brooklyn Museum and held an event with over 100 people attending. We have also had success in doing offsite events at the Aquarium at Coney Island.

Lebanon, NH: Everyone LOVES LOVES LOVES having student volunteers! My sorority sisters from Dartmouth College come every month, usually 10-15 at a time. This has been an enormously successful part of our Café – both sides enjoy interacting with each other, and it enhances the socialization portions of our program. I could go on and on, and feel free to ask questions, but I'll leave it there for now.

• Any good changes you've made?
Lebanon, NH: We didn't start with student volunteers; that came after 3 months of the program and realizing that we could use some more help. We also moved to a new location in May 2012 (after starting in January 2011) because we outgrew our old space. We now often have nearly 70 attendees (40+ guests, entertainment groups, and volunteers)

Erie, NY: The agenda: a mix of activities including memory games, crafts, exercise, old trivia that we do together, Tai Chi, music, Bingo (we cheat so the care receivers & caregivers win, not the volunteers), beanbag toss, have a golf tee, 'What's in the Sock?' game, etc. We don't do the same things every month.

- Everyone loves the *Prize Basket*, filled with small donated items, some from health fairs, etc. Bingo winners often select a "kids" item to take home to a grandchild.

- Being flexible and sensitive to the needs of the people attending. Some (care receivers) men just want to sit and talk, we have a retired judge and a professor who don't enjoy physical activities, but get into word games (with a volunteer discreetly joining in) and visiting with each other. Other men love the bean bag toss and get a rousing game going, including cheerleaders (usually the volunteers.)

- Encouraging the women caregivers to do things with each other – they really appreciate the crafts – and we've seen them exchanging recipes and helpful tips.

Minneapolis, MN: Meeting twice month at 1-3 pm after lunch and before dinner, yet many come and buy lunch and eat during our meeting as well while others eat snacks.

Richardson, TX: Our simple icebreaker: introductions at the start of each meeting, has worked well to get our meetings started. A simple guided project (making Valentine's Day cards with rubber stamps & glitter glue was enjoyed by all). It's also fun to share when members bring their artwork, woodworking projects or other hobby items.

Sacramento, CA: My group loves games, so I invent silly games that test eye-hand coordination. Latest was one I saw at the park called 'washers.' You toss a washer toward the circles on a board marked 5, 4, 3, etc. You have to get 10 points to win. They also loved pin-the-green-toupee on the paddy raccoon so he can go celebrate St Paddy's (a version of pin-the-tail on the donkey). Getting my group to perform, take pictures, make stuff for me (one caregiver made a great donation jar) AND thereby OWN their own Café.

Asheville, NC: We involved the leaders of the three church cafés in Asheville on the planning team for the conference, *The Sacred Journey of Dementia* (which was not a religious focus, but a focus on our common humanity.) It was a fantastic experience, great team – though I was the only person who knew them all. We had a Memory Café all day at the conference, and used the volunteers from those three churches Memory Café leadership teams to host the conference café as well as be volunteers for other aspects of the conference. It built a real community of those who were growing in their compassion and knowledge about dementia.

• Problems you've had?

Asheville, NC: MARKETING! Although we have had wonderful attendance at 4 of the 5 café, (the cafés at the churches have the best and most loyal attendance) we know there are many more people out there who would enjoy this, if they just learn about it. It's a challenge. We live in an area known to be a draw for retirees, so we have the population, but the cafés are run by volunteers who don't have any marketing experience. They are faithful to the event, but could use help with easy ways to do outreach. Also most volunteers are seniors themselves, trying to reach out to seniors, so the social media network is not well used by any of the above.

Lebanon, NH: Just the space issue, really. Plus, the students are on break for 2-3 meetings a year. The guests definitely miss the students when they are gone!

Minneapolis, MN: None at all. Everyone is so appreciative. They tell us all the time, if the get-together was offered every day, they would come!

Erie, NY: Low attendance. We miss our "regulars" when they no longer attend as they've moved on to a higher level of care or have scheduling conflicts with their adult day program. Caregivers want nice crafts, not childish throw-away things. It's a challenge to make it work for both the caregiver and care receiver and not cost much. Sometimes it works well when volunteers help care receivers with the crafts one-on-one and the caregivers have fun on their own. The caregivers don't think twice about what their loved ones are doing, they are confident he/she is having a good time. We use more volunteers than we originally anticipated. Both the caregivers and care receivers like the attention and appreciate direction, companionship and encouragement.

Richardson, TX: We haven't had much success in getting volunteers to assume leadership of the group, even in our most successful Café. The original team that developed the Café cannot continue to facilitate every meeting and we're not yet sure how we will solve this issue.

Sacramento, CA: Homeless guy keeps trying to 'help me.' I let him help till guest arrive. Then I say come back at 4pm and make a plate of food, after the guests have eaten.

Bill peed on him himself and his wife was embarrassed. Not a problem for me, but I said "hey," – he wandered away and did it out of sight, pretty good! and pants dried fast...told her we are all here for her and Bill.

- **Anything else you'd like us to pass along?**

Asheville, NC: We plan to bring the memory café teams together in the fall for a 'kick-off' to get everyone re-energized for the new year – fall, winter, spring. – in order to continue to cultivate and develop teams of people in the community who are dealing with people with dementia in a new and more respectful way.

Because I feel so strongly that those with a diagnosis need more advocacy, I included in a grant request a little funding to hold a conference that would give those with a diagnosis, a role in leadership in planning the conference and in presenting at the conference. We planned a conference that ended up having 200 people attend and received rave reviews. Many told us that the day changed their lives as they had not had an experience of hearing from those with a diagnosis. At the opening we showed 'Cannan & James' Story.' James has a diagnosis and Cannan is his caregiver. It framed the day. We also had a panel of people with a diagnosis, from our Early Memory Loss Collaborative Group in the afternoon.

In addition to 'Cannan & James' Story' we showed 'Please Talk With Us Not About Us.' This phrase came from people in our support group who're tired of going to conferences on dementia to be talked 'about.' They speak about being humiliated. They want to be included in the conversation and to be resources, not just the objects of all the dread. When presenters try to push thru the wall of fear of the attendees, they often objectify people with dementia in their role-playing.

Erie, NY: Most of the care receivers attending our Memory Café are male – not what we expected – so we need keep that in mind as we plan the agenda.

Albuquerque, NM: Our emphasis is fourfold: physical exercise, mental exercise, vascular health, and social interaction in some form or other most meetings. We have 15 minutes of singing from an outside source, some joint singing of familiar songs, a trip down memory lane, some objects of the past to rekindle thought and conversation, a time of "what was good this month" so both caregiver and person with dementia can participate if they desire, and some videos that go along with a topic that is being or has been discussed. Trying to find a good balance to serve both caregiver and their loved ones is a goal for us. Upcoming topics include chair yoga, a short conversation with a speech and language pathologist, an afternoon in "Texas" with songs and videos of that state, and an afternoon with therapy dogs.

Dover Study Synopsis

A study certified by Keene State College, NH

For the full survey, go to:
alzheimers–cafe–report–2015–web.pdf

Location: THE CHILDREN'S MUSEUM OF NEW HAMPSHIRE

What we studied

The primary objective of the study was to determine if our Café was perceived to be beneficial by those who attend. We also wanted to identify specific benefits, and learn what improvements could be made, based on participants' views. As research is limited, we hoped to add to the body of knowledge regarding this community-based, non-pharmacological approach to supporting people affected by dementias, their family and friends. Finally, we anticipated that armed with data indicating the benefits of an Alzheimer's Café, more Cafés would emerge for families to visit.

> **"I made some new friends. That's a great thing – I got to understand the progression of Alzheimer's in various stages. It gives me a better understanding."**
>
> – Café Attendee

The Tools We Used

Observations:

Indications of wellbeing included shaking hands, patting someone's back, and nodding good-bye or engaging in other socially acceptable ways. Indications of feeling pleasure, sustaining attention, and showing interest and self-esteem were also observed most of the time. Sadness or negative affect (agitation or anger) was rarely observed.

Questionnaires:

All of the care partners agreed that since attending the café they found new resources, felt more relaxed and were more involved in the community. The majority (90%) agrees that they feel happier after attending the Café. Some drove up to 35 miles to attend the café; the average was 10.4 miles. Two participants with dementia completed the questionnaire and both agreed that they feel more relaxed and happier after attending the Café.

Interviews:

Attendees stated, "It makes me happier." When asked if they would recommend attending the café to others, they responded, "Yes, because there are people like me." Care partners like the friendship at the Café, and that it's an outing that both partners enjoy. They like seeing their loved ones happy, meeting other people and learning from others' experiences. They also enjoy being socially engaged and building a community. Several care partners expressed concern that the Café was becoming too crowded and noisy. They unanimously said they'd recommend attending the Café to others because it's " cheerful, welcoming, and friendly".

What We Learned

Several common themes emerged across the various data collecting methods about the perceived benefits of attending an Alzheimer's Café. The Café is perceived as a fun, relaxed place that promotes a sense of normalcy, a non-judgmental environment where both care partners feel happier and find a strong sense of connectedness to others and to a community. The same relaxed feeling was reported by staff and volunteers who share the observation that the Café is a place where care partners find an opportunity to relax and feel happiness at seeing their loved one happy. Significantly, unanimous whole-hearted agreement came from both partners who say they would recommend the café to others.

One notable finding is that people with dementia reported that what they liked about coming to the Café was seeing "familiar" and "good" faces. Despite the short-term memory loss associated with dementia, repeated visits with people whom they have seen before seems to have a positive effect. Those who attend often seem to feel a sense of inclusion and camaraderie.

> **"Some of the good things that have happened since coming to the Café are the building up of community and learning about different people and what they do. I like seeing the happiness of the person I'm caring for, seeing them comfortable and not afraid; keeping alive those cognitive skills is important."**
>
> **– Café Attendee**

Volunteers – A qualitative analysis of the responses revealed common themes of enjoyment at seeing attendees feeling content and happy and creating new friendships. The volunteers especially like the nonjudgmental feeling of the café, and that most attendees smile a lot and seem relaxed. They also feel good about learning more about Alzheimer's and being able to help the families who attend the Café. Volunteers said they'd like to have music or other entertainment more often at the Café.

> **"We always tell people about the Café. I think it is very important that both patient [sic] and caregiver have an outlet to be with other people. It is somewhat comforting to know you are not alone."**
>
> **– Café Attendee**

Conclusion

The social, person-to-person encounters at the Alzheimer's Café generate a feeling of well-being and contentment for both partners, and can renew and strengthen their relationships with other people at a time when connections are fading. We encourage others to replicate this non-medication, non-invasive, low-cost approach that can benefit people with Alzheimer's disease and their care partners. It is our hope that by sharing these evaluation results, more café s will be established, more care partners will attend, and more families will experience a measure of respite from the inevitable march of the disease.

> **"The Café is gentle. It is a place to solve problems. The #1 requirement is to show up."**
>
> **– Café Attendee**

Boston Study Synopsis

The Memory Café at JF&CS in Boston is fortunate to have the involvement of student volunteers, who have received dementia/Alzheimer's training.

In 2015, the coordinator Beth Soltzberg decided to join forces with nearby colleges and other organizations to survey the benefits and satisfaction of volunteers and participants at her café.

Participants, half of whom have attended at least five times. Comments from a couple of participants:

> "I like the attitude that Beth sets at the Café which is supportive, friendly, encouraging and non competitive "

> "An opportunity in a safe and non-judgmental environment for socialization with other memory impaired individuals and their caregivers on a regular basis."

How to improve the café:
One respondent had two requests: open talk about dementia and healthier snacks, fruits rather than pastries.
Another requested information on technology to improve motional states: light therapy exercise, entertainment, and relaxation; interactive computer games for physical movement and exercise customized music playlists.

Activities that people enjoyed:
An art project, a singalong, a dance program, a discussion or a game that includes the participation of most people.

What people did not like:
Passive programs, such as watching a movie, even a favorite like "My Fair Lady"

The Volunteers
83% of volunteers are from Brandeis Lab and University, and Waltham Group
50% of all volunteers have participated 5 or more times
50% participated 1 or 2 times

What was liked best
"I loved meeting the elders and hearing their stories"

What was liked least.
Some mentioned activities taking over with no time left for conversations and interactions. Presentations not being interactive enough.

Changes and improvements
More chances to interact and having more engaging activities. The volunteers describe the Café as a rare opportunity to bring together people who would otherwise rarely interact.

National Questionnaire 2015

In late 2015, we sent questionnaires to all the cafes with whom we had email contact and had responses from 38 dyads of care partner attendees (total 72) and 8 café leaders.

Eight café leaders responded. One of the respondent is on the leadership team of a cluster of 20 cafés.

Locations: Five cafés take place at community venues, museums, cafés, and libraries; two at a senior center and one in a private garden.

Advantages to current venues: Accessible, easy to find, and familiar; handicapped accessible. cheerful, and neutral ground. No marketing pressure, which could happen at a senior community. None of the respondents pay rent, plenty of free parking; An additional comment: *it's a museum, so it is interesting.*

Disadvantages: Three leaders mentioned disadvantages to their particular venues: Distance from the parking lot, seasonal outdoor venue, and restaurant can get noisy.

None of the leaders would consider changing venue.

Budgets: How do you pay for expenses?
    2 Sponsorships
    5 Solicit small donations for snacks and supplies
    1 Attendees pay for themselves (public cafes or potlucks)
Half of the leaders are volunteers. Sponsors, employers or venue pays the rest.

Two cafes are led by family members, the rest by professionals,
• Only one leader mentions being concerned about continuity

Two of the eight cafes follow the *"European Model"* a Mix of socializing and formal information/lectures. The majority follow the *"American Model"*, focused on socialization.

146

When and who started your café?
Half of the eight cafes were started in 2014 and later, two by health and senior care programs, one by a family member, and one as a project for a Masters Degree. The Texas cafes were started by a small group of professionals; by early 2016, there are almost two dozen cafe in the central Texas region.

None of the cafes offer respite care (where you can leave your elder while you take time off. All the cafes expect caregivers/companions/families to stay. The exception is for participants living with younger onset/early stage dementia, who are still mostly independent. None of the cafes screen their participants, except the "garden" venue, which screens for safety reasons.

What has worked particularly well?
• Live music outdoors in the summer draws the best attendance
• Most enthusiastic response was to therapy dog visits.
• Appointing one of the participant couples as communications directors and having them send out an email reminder every month.

Problems you've had?
• Attendance is erratic, sometimes 11, sometimes 2.
• We're off to a slow start but it's picking up!
• I wouldn't do anything differently. Word is getting out and things are picking up.

Anything else you'd like us to pass along to our readers
• You don't need a lot of food. Our café is held at 2 pm; people tend to eat 1 cookie and have a drink and that's it.
• For publicity, concentrate on word of mouth through agencies for the elderly and people with Alzheimer's.
• Need a group of committed participants for the first 6 months.
• Remind support groups of times and locations of the cafes.
• We noticed very little of the refreshments were being consumed. Switched to easy-to-handle items, e.g., drinks in cups so people don't have to open screw-cap bottles.

Participants' Responses

(Totally subjective and unscientific)
We had responses from 38 dyads (total around 76)
Average of number of café sessions attended: 16.
Average distance traveled: 8.5 miles (up to 45 miles)
Most stay for the duration of the two-hour café.

We ranked preferences of activities:

Caregivers or family members listed as their top choices:
Sharing resources, connecting, conversations, relaxing, and being comfortable.
They also liked the art projects and music performances.

Attendees living with Alzheimer's/dementia had slightly different reactions.
Connecting with others in similar situations topped their list. Next: Sing-alongs, followed by jokes, storytelling and conversations. Music performers, snacks, feeling safe and comfortable in public, and getting back to the core of their relationship.

What would you like to see more of at your café?
"More conversation. Interaction. Music. Games."

Is there anything that bothers you-at the café?
"Not much. Some activities too advanced for cognitive skills"

What are some positive things the café?
"Being included in activities."
"Getting out to do something different"
"Mom and I really love it. Miss it when we can't make it."
"Stress relief. Laughter. Joy"
"Knowing we're not alone with Alzheimer's"
"Mom doesn't care what we do. She's just happy to get out"

Educational programs and formal presentations by experts on Alzheimer's/dementia were listed near the bottom of priorities.

Chapter Eleven

Bioclinica Clinical Trials

"Thank you to Bioclinica and its Patient Recruitment-Retention services team for their support in the development of this book."
                                                                Jytte Lokvig

I.   Why are clinical trials important for those with Alzheimer's disease?

Clinical trials are especially important for those living with Alzheimer's disease because there is currently no known treatment for halting the progression of the disease. Fortunately, there is exciting research in progress around the world that could lead to more effective treatment options. By participating in a clinical trial, patients could potentially gain access to cutting-edge medical treatments that could help them manage their symptoms and prolong their quality of life. There are a few reasons why someone living with Alzheimer's disease might consider participating in a clinical trial.

For themselves

Since there is no surefire way to prevent Alzheimer's progression, people are often motivated to try new things in an effort to find something that might help them better manage their symptoms. By participating in a clinical trial, they could gain access to potentially beneficial medical treatments. They could also benefit from the thorough and professional medical care associated with their participation in the clinical research study. This care is usually free of charge. Many participants also value the sense of community, and the chance to learn more about their disease.

According to some studies, people who participate in Alzheimer's clinical trials are less likely to be placed in a nursing home than those who do not[1]. This is an important goal for many – to live at home for as long as possible.

For their families

The causes of Alzheimer's disease are not completely understood, thus, clinical research is particularly important so we can better understand the way the disease works, and how to treat it. Without these studies, we are unable to determine if a potential new medication is effective and safe. By participating in a clinical trial, people are not only helping themselves – they are helping future generations.

For society

Alzheimer's disease affects one in eight Americans, and it is the sixth leading cause of death in the United States. It also costs the US medical system billions of dollars per year. Often, people who participate in clinical trials are motivated by a sense of altruism. It is a chance to give back to the community by furthering the advancement of medicine and science.

Clinical research allows you to play an active role in the fight against Alzheimer's disease, and in your own medical care.

II.   What is a clinical trial?

Ninety percent of what we know about Alzheimer's disease has been discovered in the last 15 years[2]. Clinical research studies, and their participants, have played a crucial part in these advancements. Unfortunately, there are a lot of misconceptions about clinical research studies, and many people don't fully understand how they work, or just how vital they are to the advancement of medicine. Let's take a closer look at clinical trials and examine the important role they play in Alzheimer's disease treatment.

Clinical research studies, also called clinical trials, allow us to study the safety and effectiveness of potential new medical treatments. They are the key to uncovering treatment advances for medical conditions, such as Alzheimer's disease. Without them, we would have no new, government-approved medical treatments on the market.

Each clinical trial has its own guidelines, known as the protocol, for the design of the study, including specific criteria for who may participate in the study. In order to ensure the safety and wellbeing of those who enroll, all study protocols must be approved by an Independent Review Board (IRB) or Ethics Committee (EC) prior to starting the study. The IRB or EC oversees the study until it is completed.

How does it work?

Depending on the type of study, patients may receive an investigational medicine, a standard or commonly-used treatment or medicine, or a "placebo." A placebo is a pill, injection, or other type of treatment that does not contain any active medicine.

In some studies, neither the participants nor the study doctors know whether or not an individual is receiving the investigational treatment or the placebo—this type of study is known as a "double-blind" study. In double-blind studies, participants are typically divided into groups. For example, 50 percent of participants may be placed into a group that receives the investigational therapy, while the other half of participants may be placed into a group that receives a placebo. The groups are determined randomly and anonymously, so there is an equal chance for everyone in the study to receive either the study drug or the placebo.

In other studies, all participants receive the investigational medication, and both the participants and the study doctors know that everyone is receiving the study drug. These are called "open-label" studies.

What is it like to be in a study?

Every study is different, just as every person is different. Each participant will have a different overall experience in a study. However, there are some common aspects of most studies.

Typically, potential study participants will:

- Complete a pre-screening questionnaire to determine pre-qualification, as determined by the study protocol

- Undergo more in-depth screening to confirm eligibility and participation in the study; this includes the Informed Consent process, which is when the study staff reviews with participants in detail all of the potential benefits and risks associated with study participation, as well as time commitments and other parameters or requirements

- Be required to attend a specified number of study-related appointments with the study doctor or other study staff, who may conduct physical and/or cognitive exams, inquire into the participant's general wellbeing, review any changes in medical history since the last visit, and more. Study participants may decide to withdrawal from the clinical trial at any time.

What happens to my personal data?

Information collected about participants during the course of the study, such as lab results and exam assessments, is protected and kept secure, in accordance with HIPAA and other local and national laws regarding privacy and personal health information. Participants are never identified by name to anyone other than the study center staff, as necessary.

The caregiver's role in a clinical trial

Caregivers play an especially important role in Alzheimer's disease research. Participating in a clinical trial is time-consuming, and it is often the caregiver's responsibility to drive his or her loved one to study-related visits. Fortunately, caregivers may also benefit from their loved one's participation, as they gain a new support network and have the opportunity to speak to medical professionals, and potentially other caregivers, about their concerns, questions and experiences.

III.   Who is Bioclinica?

About Bioclinica

Bioclinica is a specialty services provider that utilizes expertise and technology to create clarity in the clinical trial process. Bioclinica is organized by three business segments to deliver focused service supporting multifaceted technologies. The Medical Imaging and Biomarkers segment provides medical imaging and cardiac safety services and includes a molecular marker laboratory. The eHealth Solutions segment comprises the eClinical Solutions platform; Financial Lifecycle Solutions; Safety and Regulatory Solutions; Strategic Consulting Services; App xChange Alliances; and eHealth Cloud Services. Under the Global Clinical Research segment, Bioclinica offers a network of research sites, patient recruitment–retention services, and a post–approval research division. The Company serves more than 400 pharmaceutical, biotechnology and device organizations –

including all of the top 20 – through a network of offices in the U.S., Europe and Asia. To learn more, go to: www.bioclinica.com

Bioclinica's Patient Recruitment-Retention division enables companies to effectively recruit, engage, and retain patients for clinical trials in a timely and cost-effective manner. When Bioclinica acquired MediciGlobal, a leading patient recruitment and retention firm for over 25 years, it extended its ability to offer an extensive patient database as well as patient communities that can be tapped for quality patients, provide customized marketing programs to aid recruitment, develop best-in-class retention materials, and offer an array of tools and services to drive site performance.

Bioclinica's Patient Recruitment-Retention Services team has been making a meaningful difference to patient health for 25 years by identifying and engaging patients for clinical research studies, and by building deep and lasting connections with patients, researchers, and pharmaceutical sponsors. Bioclinica's clinical research study recruitment practices are guided by global standards and by a concern for the lives of the patients who put their trust in us. We make certain that those who participate in clinical research studies fully understand what study participation means, and ensure that their participation is guarded by strict privacy policies.

Bioclinica is an industry leader in the use of social media and internet-based technologies to connect patients with physicians and clinical research studies. We manage 40 Facebook health condition-related communities that have more than one million members and receive more than 12 million visitors weekly.

Bioclinica's Alzheimer's experience

Bioclinica has recruited patients for seven clinical research studies on Alzheimer's, encompassing more than 60 study sites with over 5,000 participants globally. Our team truly understands this disease and the affects it has on patients and their loved ones.

Bioclinica created the Facebook community *Alzheimer's Team,* an engaged online community with over 1.5 million visitors per week, and more than 273,000 members. In the U.S., the *Alzheimer's Team* Facebook community has been instrumental in filling the previously un-met need of connecting Alzheimer's caregivers through advocacy, word-of-mouth, and online support. Bioclinica also manages *Alzheimer's Team Hispanic,* a Facebook community with almost 13,000 members, and *Alzheimer's Research,* a Facebook community where people living with Alzheimer's can find support and resources, and make connections.

IV. How can I get involved in an Alzheimer's clinical study?

If you or a loved one are interested in learning more about a clinical study in your area, visit clinicaltrials.gov. This website lists all legitimate, approved clinical research studies for all conditions, including Alzheimer's.

Finding a sense of community is so important for people living with Alzheimer's, and for their loved ones. We are pleased and proud to have played a role in creating this book, an important resource for those looking to learn more about Alzheimer's Cafés.

Resources

For an expanded list of resources, go to: www.alzheimersatoz.com

Dr. Jytte Lokvig
    Websites: www.alzheimersatoz.com
        The National Registry of Alzheimer's and Memory Cafes:
        www. AlzheimersCafe.com
    Facebook Pages:
        Alzheimer's A to Z
        Alzheimer's Café
    Books by Dr. Jytte Lokvig
        Alzheimer's A to Z, ISBN 978-1572243958
        Alzheimer's Creativity Project, ISBN 978-0971039025

Bioclinica
    Websites: www.bioclinica.com
    www.clinicaltrials.gov
    www.healthcommunities.com/alzheimers-disease
    Facebook Page:
        Alzheimer's Team

Alzheimer's and Related Dementia:
    Alzheimer's Disease Education and Referral (ADEAR)
        https://www.nia.nih.gov/alzheimers
    Alzheimer's Association: www.alz.org
    National Parkinson Foundation: www.parkinson.org
    Association for Frontotemporal Degeneration:
        www.theaftd.org
    Lewy Body Dementia Association: www.lbda.org

Messages from people living with dementia:

Richard Taylor, PhD
    Alzheimer's From the Inside Out, ISBN: 978-1932529233
    Be with me TODAY, DVD: haveagoodlife.com

Kate Swaffer
    What the hell happened to my brain? ISBN-10:1849056083
    The Power of Language YouTube: Kate Swaffer

David Kramer, MD.
    Facebook Page: *Living Well with Alzheimer's*
    YouTube: David Kramer, MD. on living well with Alzheimer's

DVD: *I Remember Better When I Paint*:
    Treating Alzheimer's through the Creative Arts
    ASIN: B002UZE8S8

DVD: Dan Cohen *Alive Inside:* ASIN: B00OPCF3EW

Creativity, Activity and Program Ideas:
    Creativity: www.alzcreativity.com
    The Alzheimer's Poetry Project: www.alzpoetry.com
    Art Therapy: www.ImStillHere.org
    Dance: www.kairosalive.org
    Museum programs: www.OpenDoorsToMemory.org
    Music: www.MusicandMemory.org

Other Good Resources:
Bathing Without a Battle: Book and DVD
   www.bathingwithoutabattle.unc.edu
Teepa Snow, www.teepasnow.com

Memory Café Catalyst, www.memorycafecatalyst.org
   An online community for organizers of memory cafés

Books by Dr. Bill Thomas:
   Second Wind: Navigating the Passage to a Slower, Deeper,
   and More Connected Life, 978-1451667578
   What Are Old People For?:
   How Elders Will Save the World, ISBN: 978-1889242200
   In the Arms of Elders: A Parable of Wise Leadership and
   Community Building, ISBN: 978-1889242101

Books by Dr. G. Allen Power, MD:
   Dementia Beyond Disease: ISBN: 978-1938870132
   Dementia Beyond Drugs: ISBN: 978-1932529562

Books by Gary Glazner
   Sparking Memories: The Alzheimer's Poetry Project
   ISBN: 978-0976260301
   Dementia Arts: ISBN: 978-1938870118

Facebook:
   Momentia Seattle
   Alzheimer's Speaks Radio
   Dementia Action Alliance USA
   Dementia Alliance International

CPSIA information can be obtained
at www.ICGtesting.com
Printed in the USA
BVOW11s2122120716

455014BV00001B/1/P